WHAT MY PATIENTS SAY

Freedom Health Centers lives up to its name. My knees were so bad I was finally considering a replacement. Freedom Health came up with a treatment plan and in about four weeks, I was walking without braces or cane and didn't need my walker at home. Now six months later, my knees feel twenty-five years younger … no pain! Best money I've spent on myself!

    I recommend everyone try Freedom Health first before taking that risky surgery!

—**Audrey E.**

Life-saving—that is not an exaggeration. I came to Freedom Health Centers for physical therapy. They are awesome, but what I got was a full, comprehensive health plan. I've lost twenty-seven pounds in about forty days. My endocrinologist has told me to stop taking my insulin. The chiropractic care, the medical professionals, weight loss team, physical therapy, massage therapists, the receptionists, billing department … everything is just awesome. Top notch … I don't have any complaints. I highly recommend this place.

—**Mr. D.P.**

Being diagnosed with autoimmune arthritis at twenty-six years old was life-changing and has been debilitating at times. I have been able to manage it fairly well while learning to deal with the pain and did not know I could live with more mobility and little to zero pain. Now after having participated in multiple areas of the clinic and working with all the staff, I feel better than ever, and I am working toward strength building rather than just trying to maintain a normal life with chronic pain. Freedom Health Centers of McKinney has been a godsend and dramatically changed my life for the better.

—**Crystal Cope**

I have worked for large hospital organizations for many years, and they have attempted to provide patient integrated treatment to no avail. The Freedom Health team has the secret sauce! I have suffered thirty-two years with an old sports injury with numerous rehab therapy attempts over the years. My sports injury had become extremely complex and affected many areas. I was a "hot mess" when I first walked in fifteen visits ago. But the Freedom Health team worked together to break it down into parts and started to work. They already have my pain at a bare minimum at worst (wondering what I'm going to do with my remaining thirteen visits? Maybe eat bonbons, LOL) and localized.

In addition, the tools they are providing me to strengthen around those problem areas are critical for me to ensure the pain doesn't return in the future (of course, I know I need to continue on the journey to keeping healthy and well) but they are teaching me and giving me everything I need to succeed. Plus, I have to mention how knowledgeable they are—my own doctors couldn't even diagnose me for years! This team not only diagnosed me and treats me, but when I come in, they know exactly where I hurt without me even telling them! They are amazing. Love, love, love them! They have truly changed my life!

—**Sherri Beasley**

Dr. Todd Molski is an incredible doctor in a league of his own. He has truly given me my life back! I found him after struggling with chronic fatigue. Some days I could not walk because my legs had zero strength for nearly ten years. I was overweight after having four children and struggled to lose the weight. Other doctors were telling me to "just eat less," except I don't eat much anyway, so they blamed my hormones. I also began to have hip and knee problems, and in my mid-forties everything seemed off. I needed serious help and not by taking drugs.

Dr. Molski's full-body exam, his bedside manner, and the genuine care he provides is second to none! He put together a plan for me and has continued to encourage me every step of the way. With his adjustments, muscle release technique for my hip and knee, and his physical therapy program, my hip and knee pain are gone. I followed his weight loss program and lost twenty-seven pounds within seven weeks, and I am continuing to work on gaining my body back—even my clarity of thinking has sharpened!

My chronic fatigue has been put to rest, and I have more energy now than I did over fifteen years ago! Dr. Molski has transformed my life and continues to walk my journey of recovery with me. It's not a magic switch or button, it's a process, and Dr. Molski is dedicated to helping me achieve my goal of living healthy, living with energy, and being there for my family for many years to come!

—**Shannon Sweat**

As a family that has experienced the failure of traditional medicine in an up close and personal way, Dr. Molski's clinic is a breath of fresh air. Our family has been blessed to be both patients and friends of Dr. Molski and have experienced first-hand the benefits of his system of care at Freedom Health Centers. The team at FHC takes health care to a new level. Call and get an appointment. Follow their instructions. Invest in yourself. We did, and we are better off for it. Thanks, Dr. Molski!

—**Joel Scrivner**

I came to Freedom Health Centers (FHC) because of debilitating daily headaches I'd had for almost two months. Regular chiropractic adjustments were not helping. What I got here was a plan and a team to not only to help get me out of pain, but to teach me how to stay out of pain if I actually applied what they taught me. I've had no headaches that last more than a few minutes since the first treatment. Sometimes headaches start to come on, but because I use the tools I've learned, they quickly subside. I'm very impressed with the intercommunication among my health team. I feel like they care enough to listen and to immediately pass the information along to the next department/team member. I feel heard, not like I'm just a part of the herd. (No more having to explain your symptoms every, single time you are passed from one team member to the next). If you want a place where you feel like your health matters as much to them as it does to you, I recommend FHC. The entire team and staff have earned my five great, big stars!

—LaRue Epler

I salute Dr. Todd Molski's vision and direction for the Freedom Heath Centers (FHC). Possibly, the concept of including all aspects of physical well-being into one environment is simple in nature but it is evolutionary in practice.

As a couple who enjoys to travel, my wife and I look forward to seeing the growth of that concept across the country. We found Freedom Health and Dr. Molski while my wife was having knee problems and deliberating about having a knee surgery, which happened to be about a year after a car accident we had been in. From the beginning, the amount of medical information shared with us in plain, understandable language and examples was simply amazing.

In addition to trying to resolve my wife's knee issue, I went because of headaches I had been having since the car accident. That is when the amazing things really started occurring.

Normally when getting chiropractic or medical help of any kind, you're called in and the doctor will tell you in medical jargon and then try to tell you in layman's terms what is going on and what they want to do to treat it. That is what happened at Freedom as well, but when the treatments actually started, the professionals there discussed every aspect of everything we were doing from body interaction with platelet-rich plasma injections (PRP) and stem cell treatment to what the physical therapy exercises we were doing were for and how they could improve our long-term outlook and how we could do them at home to heal and correct our own bodies on an ongoing basis.

My wife's knee has not been a problem since her treatment, and my daily to multiple times a week headaches have vanished. Since then we have taken advantage of other well-being services including the wellness training and nutrition options to produce significant improvement in weight loss and blood pressure. My pre-treatment was moderate hypertensive (160/90 range), and the last check after workout was 122/72. My wife, who is on blood pressure medication, went from 140/90 to 120/70 range as well. Again both of those are from a combination of the wellness training and weight loss programs offered and monitored by the Freedom Health professionals.

These people are amazing! When we travel there are times we need to get an adjustment due to bad hotel pillows etc., and we've been fortunate to find well-qualified care in multiple places; some with additional services such as therapy or massages, but none with the full gamut of services that Dr. Todd has put together at his FHC.

When we discuss the FHC concept with the professionals in other places, they are always blown away that someone has put that much skill and multiple professions under one roof to develop a full-body plan to help each individual. We always assure them it is real and not something we made up.

Also, everyone who walks into FHC is treated as an individual when there, and it seems like every one of those helpful doctors, nurses, and therapists know exactly what your particular ailment is, and how they can best treat you and empower you to help yourself do it, too.

Simply put, we have traveled the country from end to end and have never seen anything like the FHC that Dr. Molski has put together. Great job, Dr. Todd!

—Larry and Dale Costello

FREEDOM

FREEDOM

THE BRAIN, BODY, GUT REVOLUTION FOR A PAIN-FREE LIFE

DR. TODD A. MOLSKI, D.C.

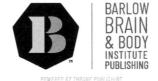

Copyright © 2022 by Dr. Todd A. Molski, D.C.

ISBN Softcover: 978-1-949550-74-0
Ebook ISBN: 978-1-949550-75-7

All rights reserved. No part of this book may be reproduced or transmitted in any form or by any means, electronic or mechanical, including photocopying, recording or by any information storage and retrieval system, without permission in writing from the copyright owner. For information on distribution rights, royalties, derivative works or licensing opportunities on behalf of this content or work, please contact the publisher at the address below.

Printed in the United States of America.

Cover Design: Mila Book Designs

Although the author and publisher have made every effort to ensure that the information and advice in this book was correct and accurate at press time, the author and publisher do not assume and hereby disclaim any liability to any party for any loss, damage, or disruption caused from acting upon the information in this book or by errors or omissions, whether such errors or omissions result from negligence, accident, or any other cause.

Barlow Brain & Body Institute
266 County Road 506
Shannon, MS 38868
www.barlowbrainandbody.com

DEDICATION

Wow! There are so many people I want to thank. I know I won't be able to get to everyone, so forgive me if I don't.

First, I have to thank my Lord and Savior, Jesus Christ. I gave Freedom Health Centers to You and You have made it a place of Mark 16:17–18. I am honored to steward it for You.

To all my staff past and present at Freedom Health Centers, teamwork makes the dream work! Special thanks to my right arm and clinic "mom," Christina Newman. You are why this clinic is the place it is. Thank you for your wisdom, for being a sounding board, and for being the blessing you are. Being a Godly woman these days is difficult, but you are a role model. Thank you for everything you are and everything you do. Another special thank you to Dr. Scott Wright. You have stuck it out with me through the ups and downs. You are a great doctor and an outstanding human being. Go Bills!

To my parents, Albert and Kathleen Molski. Thanks, Mom, for all the advice, all the help, all times you were there for me. I can never repay that. Thank you, Dad, for being a great role model. I wish I could talk to you right now, Dad, to share this book with you. I know you would be proud. I will talk to you soon, but for now I have work to do here. Save me a seat in heaven. I love you both more than you will ever know. Thank you for making me the man I am.

Lastly, to my wife, Katrina Molski, the love of my life. God put us together, and I am so grateful. Your love, your understanding, your advice, your kindness, your organization skills (they are incredible!), and your ability to put up with all my craziness has sustained me and given me the biggest blessing in my life. I could not have done this without you. Thank you for being there for me through it all. I can't wait to see where God brings us in this next season of our lives. You mean more to me than you will ever know. Thank you from the bottom of my heart.

TABLE OF CONTENTS

Foreword xv

PART ONE: Shared Philosophy 1

Chapter One: Chiropractic Called Me 3

Chapter Two: A Winning Team 13

Chapter Three: There's More Below the Surface 17

PART TWO: Shared Understanding 21

Chapter Four: Untangling the Web of Dysfunction 23

Chapter Five: Key 1 – Oxygen 27

Chapter Six: Key 2 – Glucose 33

Chapter Seven: Key 3 – Stimulation 39

Chapter Eight: Key 4 – Autoimmune Disorders 45

Chapter Nine: Key 5 – Inflammation 51

Chapter Ten: Key 6 – Neurotoxins 57

Chapter Eleven: Key 7 – The Brain-Gut Connection 61

PART THREE: Shared Follow Through 69

Chapter Twelve: How Exams Help You Heal. 71

Chapter Thirteen: Our Program 77

Chapter Fourteen: A Positive Outcome Is Our Goal 83

FOREWORD

Sixteen years ago, I had no idea what I was getting into. I was a frustrated mom in need of help for my teenage son. Medical professionals offered little hope for a "fix" to the issues we faced. Friends of ours, who spent time agreeing in prayer with us to find a solution, spotted a poster while visiting Dr. Molski's office. They told me about Dr. Molski, and we made an appointment. The office was warm and welcoming. The staff assured me that Dr. Molski was the answer to our problems—they had no idea how right they were.

I quickly learned that Dr. Molski didn't claim to have all the answers but worked diligently to find every solution. He brought the leadership skills he gained from his team sports days to the office and partnered with both his staff and his patients.

His mission has always been to bring true healthcare to his community. This resonated with me, and I wanted to join his team. Not only did I have the privilege of joining his team, but I became an expert in managing his unique flagship office.

Dr. Molski's pursuit of greater knowledge of the workings of the human body and how to make it more efficient was contagious. He invested in me and helped me become a Certified Physician Practice Manager. Dr. Molski is a fabulous teacher. His knowledge and guidance will help your body work in the way the Creator designed. You've made the right choice reading *Freedom*. Through this book, you'll be able to easily identify areas that you need to be evaluated.

No matter where you are in this journey, this book will give you the information to confidently move forward to freedom—freedom from pain, freedom from limited movement, and freedom to enjoy your life!

Christina Newman, CPPM

PART ONE

SHARED PHILOSOPHY

1

CHIROPRACTIC CALLED ME

I was only trying to get out of bed.
Why did it suddenly feel like someone was stabbing me with a hot knife between my shoulder blades?

I was fourteen years old and an athlete. Of course, I had experienced pain before—but this was different. I hadn't fallen and scraped my knee. There was no ankle sprain or fractured collarbone like I had witnessed with some of the other players on my soccer team. I couldn't make sense of the pain I was experiencing. I thought if I just stayed still, the unbearable stabbing pain would just go away. When my naive tactics failed to work, panic took control and I yelled for my mom.

Before I was born, my mom had been in a terrible car accident, so she was no stranger to excruciating pain. I remember hearing stories about all the pain medications she had been prescribed because of her injuries. They prevented her from even making a successful trip down the stairs in our home without help. After weeks of enduring the effects of traditional pain "management," she resorted to a less traditional approach and sought relief on the table of a chiropractor.

According to my dad, after the first couple of adjustments, it was like a veil had been lifted. Within two weeks of chiropractic treatment, my mom had full range of motion, no pain, and was able to get off all pain medications. While it is hard for me to imagine my mother going through such a painful experience, I am grateful that she did; it prompted her to take me to the chiropractor when I was fourteen and could barely move. After one week of seeing the chiropractor, the stabbing pain stopped and has never returned.

Although there had not been a direct correlation to an injury, the stabbing sensation I experienced between my shoulder blades was likely due to the physical stress of playing high-level competitive sports. Still, the drive and passion I had for playing soccer were stronger than the memory of the pain, and I went on to play at a collegiate level.

After a while, I started to develop painful fluid build-up on my knee. The team sports medicine doctors tried everything to relieve the pain, including a failed attempt to drain my knee with a needle. Once again, Mom came to my rescue and suggested I find a local chiropractor. Wise enough to follow her advice, I quickly made an appointment with a local sports and family chiropractor. Limping in for my first appointment, I remember not expecting I would get help with me knee. I had gotten relief when it was my back, but what could a chiropractor do to help my knee?

The chiropractor explained that everything is linked together. Just like in that old song, *Dem Bones,* "the knee bone connected to the thigh bone." I was amazed when the knee pain vanished immediately after the doctor adjusted my lower back, neck, knee, and ankle.

After the adjustments, the doctor talked to me about the daily trauma I was subjecting my body to as a collegiate-level athlete. He talked about the importance of following a maintenance care plan, so I didn't continue to find myself in pain. I am confident that my willingness to follow his recommendations and continue with regular visits for "fine-tuning" are not only the reason that I could complete that soccer season, but also a large part of why I was able to go on to have an early career as a semi-professional soccer player.

While soccer is what gave me my drive, I knew that I would have to find a major program of study for life beyond soccer. From an early age, I knew that I wanted to help people in some way and always assumed it would be in some type of medical field. Although I knew that traditional medicine was not my path, I wanted to learn everything I could about the human body and the way it works. I went into pre-med and graduated from college with a degree in biology and a minor in psychology. After graduation I knew one thing: I didn't want to go to medical school, but the question of what I was going to do with my life still remained.

• • • • •

My parents were amazing role models and showed me what could be possible with integrity, hard work, and a constant ability to keep learning. After serving in the Korean War, my dad had taken a job climbing telephone poles to repair phone lines for Southwestern Bell. Over the years, with hard work and perseverance, he worked his way up to an executive management position, and by the time I graduated from college, he had been promoted to oversee an international region with AT&T. This took my parents from St. Louis, Missouri, to Sydney, Australia, where they were living after I graduated. Unsure of my direction and purpose, I decided to spend the holidays in Sydney with my parents.

For the most part, I spent my time in Sydney seeing the sights with my mom while my dad worked. On one of our more memorable day trips, we walked around the Sydney Botanical Gardens. We stopped to look out over the Sydney Opera House and the Harbor Bridge when I turned to her and asked, "Mom, what do you think I should do with my life?"

Just as she had done for me so many times before, my mom came through with the answer. "Why don't you go to chiropractic college?" she casually suggested, as if the answer had been obvious all along. In that instant, my future started to come into focus. I thought to myself, "I could do that!"

I started to anxiously anticipate the end of the holidays so that I could return to the U. S. and pursue this new path. Four years later, I graduated with my Doctorate in Chiropractic from Logan University in St. Louis, Missouri, and immediately started my life as a chiropractor. I moved to Dallas, Texas, where I worked with a group of doctors.

Fortunately for me, while working at a clinic in East Texas, I met my wife, Katrina. The more time I spent with her, the more I knew she was the girl for me. Like me, Katrina had endured the physical consequences of her youth. As a kid, she lived on a farm where there was always a lot of work to be done in the garden or taking care of the animals, including pigs, cows, chickens, and horses. She had been thrown while on horseback twice; one time hitting her head on a rock when she fell, knocking her out and resulting in a concussion. What most people don't know is that six hours after a concussion you develop a leaky gut. It is no surprise that she had migraines, sinus issues, and gut problems from that moment on (although she was good at hiding them).

Like so many of the patients that come into my office, Katrina had tried going to chiropractors before without success, so she brushed off all chiropractors. Early on, I had to convince her to let me do what I do so I could help her. Within weeks of starting her treatments with me, we were able to eliminate her headaches and sinus infections. However, helping to heal her gut was a bigger challenge.

Three months after we were married, I opened my practice in McKinney, Texas. On the day of the grand opening, Katrina was in the hospital due to complications from a bout of food poisoning. While she was physically absent from the ceremony, she was and continues to be a huge influence in my practice. My drive to help her, and patients like her, motivates me to continuously seek more information and better tools. Ultimately, Katrina was the inspiration behind integrating the clinic (more on this later), which helps us provide better testing and treatments to support improved outcomes for our patients.

● ● ● ● ●

I learned quickly that being a chiropractor took a lot of energy and stamina. Luckily, the years I spent as an athlete provided the perfect training for the skills I would need to endure. As I look back over my path to becoming a chiropractor, I truly believe God led me into the exact experiences that would equip me to help people. For instance, as the goalkeeper in soccer, I relied heavily on quick reflexes and the strength and dexterity of my hands to catch the ball, and those same skills help me treat patients today. Each moment on my path—getting out of bed at fourteen with unbearable pain, walking with my mom through the Sydney Botanical Gardens, and meeting Katrina—were serendipitous moments that led me into a career and practice that I love.

DON'T EVER LET THE FIRE GO OUT

Working with patients for over twenty-four years in chiropractic practice might lead some to become desensitized to the miraculous healing that happens in this line of work. But that's not me. When I reflect on the things that have kept me motivated and fueled my passion, something my mom said to me in high school comes to mind: "Todd, don't ever let the fire go out."

I've lived my life by those words and after twenty-four years, I *still* wake up every morning wanting to go into the office, wanting to help people. The sometimes-miraculous nature of my patient's results isn't what keeps my fire from going out. It's the *process* we work through with each patient. The process isn't just the adjustment; it's investigating the problem, uncovering the answers, and seeking out additional ways to help our patients achieve optimal results. The fire is sparked by being a part of something bigger than just me, being a part of a team.

In all my years in sports, I was often the team captain or in other leadership roles, another way God prepared me for my future. Today, I am able to accomplish so much more with the integrated team of professionals we have assembled at my clinic. The team gives me purpose and drives me to find better ways to help patients.

One of the most important team members I had early on was my wife, Katrina. As I've said, her continuing health issues were a big factor in why we started to look into ways to grow the practice beyond chiropractic care. Another factor stemmed from some business issues we experienced in the start-up years of the clinic. In school, we are taught to be doctors, not business people. Generously, Katrina stepped away from her teaching career to help me get my business working better and more organized. In a matter of weeks, she was able to get us caught up. She then worked tirelessly to help me expand our patient services.

● ● ● ● ●

As my business entered this period of growth, the first piece we brought under our umbrella of integrated care was nutrition. In the years since, our team has grown to include a medical doctor, nurse practitioner, additional chiropractors, a rehabilitation team, a nutrition and weight loss department, wellness coaches, and a massage therapist. Our integrated efforts are also enhanced by the administrative and operational team that keeps everything running smoothly. The enjoyable environment of the clinic is made possible because our team works together, approaching each client with the best possible options and care.

When the practice finally got big enough, Katrina was able to go back to *her* calling, teaching reading and writing to elementary school kids. The practice wouldn't be what it is today without Katrina's influence. Her encouragement to grow and integrate also helped us uncover some of the issues that were causing her pre-existing gut problems. With the addition of other physicians and disciplines, we were able to provide enhanced testing, one of which revealed that Katrina was massively gluten sensitive. After working with our nutrition and wellness teams, most of her gut symptoms were eliminated. However, health is a journey. You don't just arrive at some abstract destination; you must continuously keep moving toward better health. Katrina's health journey has seen significant improvements, and those were largely made possible by the evolution of our clinic.

From my days as a team captain to now running a multi-faceted clinic, I have not let my fire go out. Rather, I have continued to fuel the fire by creating a team with the same passions and values as I do. At the top of that list is helping people.

PUTTING THE PIECES TOGETHER

In all of my years spent as an athlete on the soccer field, perhaps the largest part of what made the experience so fulfilling was being on a team; working together for the same result—to win the game. While my time on the field taught me the value of a strong team, my years spent as team captain taught me the importance of being a strong team leader. Today, I constantly aim to improve myself to be the best team leader I can be to support the clinic, the team, and the patients we see.

When I first started my practice, I was a solo chiropractor and realized quickly that I wasn't able to achieve the best results for some patients. I would treat them in my office, then they would have to go elsewhere, to their medical doctor or their physical therapist. No one was collaborating or communicating for the benefit of the patient. In fact, it was the opposite. In most cases, it felt like a turf war. When this happened, the only person who really lost was the patient. They weren't achieving the results I knew were possible. My number one priority is the patient and helping them as best I can. In order to do this, I set out to build an integrated team where the patient had their chiropractor, medical doctor, and physical therapist under the same roof. Instead of never communicating, each provider is now able to work together for the benefit of the patient.

• • • • •

Early on in my career as a solo chiropractor, a patient came to me seeking help for her new baby. The baby had a fever, but the bigger concern was that the fever would fluctuate from 99 degrees to 104 degrees, which is a dangerous spike. The doctors at the hospital decided to do a spinal tap, but, considering the extreme nature of the procedure, the mother consulted with me before moving forward. I dropped what I was doing and made my way to the hospital as quickly as I could. Walking through the sliding glass doors, I immediately felt the disapproving glares from the medical doctors. I felt like I needed those Groucho disguise glasses just to get into the hospital to help this delicate, tiny infant. The doctors didn't want to listen to what I had to say and scoffed at the alternative options I offered. Despite the doctors' resistance, the mother allowed me to conduct a non-invasive and painless adjustment on that baby. Later, the mother called to say that the fever had gone away ... *without* the involvement of a spinal tap.

● ● ● ● ●

Just like for that mother, more often than not, the burden of building a care team and of bridging the gap between providers falls on the patient or their advocate. If that mother came into our practice today, she would have had the medical doctor *and* the chiropractor collaborating under one roof to advise her toward the best possible outcome with the least invasive approach to helping her baby. There wouldn't have been any conflict that caused her additional stress and worry.

Our team focus is always on taking a deeper look into the underlying causes of the issues we treat; seeking to put the pieces of our patients' health puzzles together. We are the patient's puzzle solver! For instance, when it came to figuring out why that baby's fever was fluctuating so dangerously, I worked to put the puzzle pieces together. If the temperature in your house is going from hot to cold in drastic swings, you first want to know *why* the fluctuations are occurring. A repairman would start with the thermostat. In the case of the fever, the first thing I looked at was the body's "thermostat," the brain and nervous system. Today our clinic can conduct in-office tests that help our team pinpoint the exact problems so we can treat them more effectively than ever before.

Just like the heating system in your house has many different parts that work together, so does your body. The different parts of the body are integrated with each other. Therefore, if a patient comes in complaining about knee pain, we don't just look at their knees, we look at the whole person. While a specialist only looks at one piece of the puzzle, our team of different professionals looks at the whole complex picture, and, collectively, we treat the patient in the most efficient and natural way possible.

2

A WINNING TEAM

We care about everyone who walks through our doors. We want the best outcome for every patient, and we will do everything in our power to help them. My goal has always been to help as many people as I can, and my team enables me to do that every day. This couldn't be done without teamwork and two crucial components of any team: communication and trust. Without these two pieces, our team doesn't work.

Miscommunication leads to problems and distrust. A team is only successful if the communication among the members is clear and valuable. At Freedom Health Centers, our first goal with any patient is to communicate with them and then with the team. We start by gathering as much information as possible about the patient, the more information we have, the more we can help. That information is given to the team members who will be caring for the patient, and at every step of care, our team connects. Our patients know we care because in every interaction, test, and treatment, we have communicated the purpose and where they are in the process.

• • • • •

Early on in my career, I saw a patient who had a litany of problems. We went through the full initial exam, and at the end of our consultation, I asked her if she had any questions. She slammed her hands down on my desk and yelled, "I want out of pain right *now!*" The woman was facing chronic issues that would take time and dedication from all members of the team, herself included. It was at this moment I realized that part of building trust with a patient is a willingness to communicate the hard truths, including pointing out when there are unrealistic expectations. Our team has the knowledge that can help patients, and we will do everything we can to help them, but the goal has to be realistic for the team to be successful. We can't just snap our fingers and heal a person.

Unfortunately, that woman didn't want to hear the truth, but the experience helped me define the way my team and I interact with clients. We are here to help them along their healing journey, but it takes time, and we communicate that with patients at every step of the process. It also requires the patient to become part of the team to follow through and play their part in order to reach the goal.

● ● ● ● ●

In stark contrast to the patient mentioned above, we recently worked with an older gentleman who came to us with knee pain. His goal was to be able to enjoy at least one dance at his granddaughter's wedding, which was to take place in several months. This was a realistic goal that the entire team could get behind. During the months of care, we communicated and adjusted his plan as needed to reach his desired outcome. Everyone had the same expectations throughout the process. After his granddaughter's wedding, he told us that he didn't just dance once, he danced the night away!

● ● ● ● ●

In order for our team to be effective, our patients must trust us. It is almost impossible to establish trust if goals are unattainable and expectations and communication are unclear. Sometimes this means we have to be honest when a patient's expectations aren't in alignment with what we are realistically able to do for them. That kind of honesty can be hard to hear, but ultimately it helps to build trust in the team and the process.

We want each of our patients to experience their own version of success. For some that is dancing at their granddaughter's wedding, for others it is living without debilitating pain. The goals may be different, but for our team the goal is always to give the patient their best possible outcome. I truly believe we are saving lives every day through our teamwork, effective communication, and the trust built as a result.

WE SAVE LIVES BY ADJUSTING THE WAY PEOPLE EAT, MOVE, AND THINK

At Freedom Health Centers, our mission is to save lives by adjusting the way people eat, move, and think. I get to watch that statement play out in amazing ways every day when I walk into our office. Our success is only possible because our team operates from a set of core values that govern the way we listen and seek to understand our patients. These core values are:

- *God:* God always provides. With Him in each of our lives and as the head of this office, we will all succeed.
- *Team/Teamwork:* Teamwork allows us to multiply our talents and achieve exponential results.
- *Dependability:* We depend on each other to do our part well. We help wherever necessary, so everything runs smoothly.
- *Caring:* We treat each patient and each other with a caring spirit. We are a caring family.
- *Trustworthiness:* To engage and experience the life-changing effects of our processes, patients and staff must have trust in our system.

- *Communication:* We know that clear communication is the key to any relationship, and without clear communication we leave room for problems. Therefore, we carefully choose our words, we bring value to the conversation every time we speak.
- *Commitment:* The unwavering commitment of the staff to the Wellness lifestyle reflects the success of the office.

These values support our overall goal—to help our patients achieve greater overall health. Our body is complex, and one issue could be an indication of something else entirely. Therefore, it is essential that we look at the body as a whole and adjust the way a patient eats, moves, and thinks.

We start this process by exploring the seven key areas of health that you are about to discover in the next several chapters. If you want a life-changing experience, you have to address these seven keys. And just as the body works as a whole, these seven key areas of health all work together. You have to address each one.

Whether you are dealing with a chronic health condition or searching for a way to feel healthier and gain more energy, these seven keys will help you begin your journey.

3

THERE'S MORE BELOW THE SURFACE

TIP OF THE ICEBERG

Have you ever studied a diagram of an iceberg? From above the surface of the water, your eye can only see about 10% of the iceberg's total mass while the remaining 90% remains out of sight, lurking below the surface. An iceberg is a good metaphor for the way we should understand the total picture of our health. The symptoms we experience represent only 10–15% of the issue that is causing those obvious symptoms to appear. To understand the whole picture, uncover the web of dysfunction, and discover the path to true healing, we have to delve below the surface.

Symptoms can also be compared to the check engine light on your car. If you're on a road trip and the check engine light comes on, you're alerted to a problem with your vehicle. Would taking a piece of duct tape and covering up that check engine light solve the problem? Absolutely not, it would only prevent you from seeing the blinking light that's alerting you to a bigger issue. In fact, covering up the check engine light puts you in greater danger in the long run because what started out as a small problem will get worse and worse if you continue on your road trip and don't address the problem. Pretty soon, you're sitting on the side of the road with smoke and steam rolling out of your engine. This is what it's like when we take medication to mask our symptoms. Covering them up doesn't change the fact that there's a problem. To really figure out the issue with our car, we must go to a mechanic and have them look under the hood. To figure out the issue with our body, we need to untangle the web of dysfunction that's causing the symptom to surface.

In a car, there are a multitude of reasons why the check engine light appears. It could be a fuel issue, a spark plug issue, a battery issue, or something else entirely. Think of your health symptoms as your body's check engine light. In the same way that a check engine light comes on for a variety of reasons, our symptoms can result from a variety of health issues. This is one of the most important concepts that I teach my patients—the root cause of symptoms is different for every single person because their web of dysfunction is completely unique.

There are three main reasons why a "one size fits all" strategy does not work for solving chronic health problems. The first reason is that two people could be experiencing the same exact symptoms for completely different reasons. For example, numbness, tingling, or burning of the feet can be caused by nerve damage in the lumbar spine at the L5 vertebrae. However, it can also be caused by Type 2 diabetes or anemia. All three disorders can cause the exact same symptom for totally different reasons. To make the tangled web of dysfunction even more complicated, many of my patients have more than one root cause of their symptoms. The bottom line is that every person's health issues must be treated uniquely.

The second reason why a "one size fits all" approach doesn't work is because a doctor with preconceived notions tends to miss important clues that reveal what's really going on beneath the surface. For someone with chronic health problems, there are multiple mechanisms that can go awry and cause dysfunction, yet show up as the same kind of symptom. These mechanisms include elements like blood sugar, anemia, or destruction of the neurological pathways. If the root cause is never addressed, the correct mechanism that needs restoration and healing will never be found. Each person is a custom case. As a functional neuro-metabolic doctor, it's my job to be smart enough to look below the surface and examine the 90% that's beneath the surface.

The third reason why a "one size fits all approach" does not work for solving chronic health problems is because it tends to produce doctors that are symptom-reduction oriented rather than results oriented. As a functional neuro-medicine doctor, I want my patients to actually get better. Every time I walk into a room with a patient, I check my ego at the door because I want to solve their problems, not mask them. I am result oriented, and I am solution oriented. I'm committed to getting results for my patients, and I will exhaust all of my resources to do it. I treat each patient like a custom, one-of-a-kind 10,000 piece puzzle. When I accept a patient for care, we sit down together and start working on that puzzle until we uncover the root cause(s) and form a plan to heal them. To truly heal, we need to target and solve the core problem. We must untangle the neuro-metabolic web of dysfunction and start a journey to regeneration and wellness.

With the first three chapters as our foundation, let's go deeper by defining and then explaining the Seven Keys to healing your chronic health problems.

PART TWO

SHARED UNDERSTANDING

4

UNTANGLING THE WEB OF DYSFUNCTION

There are seven key areas of health that I look at when I'm trying to untangle someone's web of dysfunction. Depending on how they're treated, these seven keys can either foster wellness and longevity or create debilitating chronic health problems because each of these keys either adds to our health or actively takes away and destroys our health. Throughout my years of practice and study, I've discovered that any kind of disruption in these seven areas is going to cause disconnection and dysfunction (check engine light) which may eventually turn into chronic issues. When I work with a patient to help them with their chronic health problems, this is always where we begin. When these seven areas are treated well, it unleashes your body's superpower which is its ability to heal itself.

THE SEVEN KEYS

1. Oxygen: Number One of the BIG Three. It is necessary and essential for life. Anoxia (which means "without oxygen") equals death. The brain and nervous system need three elements to function at peak level, and oxygen is one of them. Oxygen is the deal breaker when it comes to neurological

health. The less oxygen we have in our bodies, the more things start to malfunction and the less capacity our bodies have to heal themselves.

2. Glucose: Number Two of the BIG Three. Glucose is your blood sugar. It's the fuel that your body needs in order to heal itself. It's also needed for the nervous system to self-regulate and function optimally. A good metaphor is that it's like the gasoline for your car engine. Cars run at a certain octane level, and if that level gets out of balance, the car isn't going to run properly. Our bodies work the same way with glucose. If there's too little, it can't function at its optimal level. If there's too much, it's not good for optimal performance either.

3. Stimulation: Number Three of the BIG Three. Stimulation is one of the main three things that the nervous system needs in order to function. The importance of stimulation can't be overstated. As Einstein once said, "Nothing happens until something moves," and in the body, no healing happens until something is stimulated. Without stimulation, the body's systems will weaken and fail. With proper stimulation, those systems will thrive and remain strong.

4. Autoimmune Disorders: Autoimmune disorders are kind of like "friendly fire." They develop when our immune system starts attacking itself instead of a foreign invader. Our immune systems should only kill the "bad guys" like viruses, but when it starts to malfunction, it doesn't just destroy antigens, it also attacks our own tissues.

5. Inflammation: Logic tells you that if your house was on fire, you wouldn't start rebuilding it until after the blazes were put out. Inflammation is like a fire in your body, and it can't start to heal until that fire is gone. True healing cannot take place until your body's inflammation is reduced.

6. Neurotoxins: These toxins are anything that's taken into the body that causes neurological damage. Unfortunately

neurotoxins are much more common that you may imagine. Table sugar is a neurotoxin. High fructose corn syrup is a neurotoxin. The artificial sweetener Aspartame is a neurotoxin. Drinking water out of a disposable plastic bottle is neurotoxic. We'll talk more in upcoming chapters about how to eliminate these harmful toxins from your life.

7. Gut Health: The role of gut health is paramount because poor gut health is a trigger for autoimmune conditions and out of control inflammatory responses. We must heal our guts in order to heal our brains and bodies. If you have a bad brain, you're guaranteed to have a bad gut too. We must restore optimal gut health and reconnect the gut-brain axis in order to achieve true healing.

While each of these seven areas are important to address individually, their true power for healing comes alive when we realize that all of these elements are interconnected. Gut health and autoimmune conditions are connected. Neurotoxins and inflammation are linked. Oxygen and stimulation are crucial to one another's roles. The body is a holistic system that must be in homeostasis in order to heal itself and function optimally. By keeping these seven primary keys in focus, your health can transform from symptom mitigation to a state of true healing and regeneration. Now that we've looked at an overview of the seven keys to optimal health, let's break each key down in greater detail.

5
KEY 1 – OXYGEN

THE ROLE OF OXYGEN

Oxygen is essential for life. This element, which makes up about 21% of the earth's atmosphere at sea level, is key to our health because our bodies need it in order to function on a cellular level. We can go without food almost forty days, and we can last about four days without water. However, we can only survive for approximately four minutes without oxygen. If the brain is deprived of oxygen for longer than that, it's a recipe for severe neurological damage and even death. Our cells need oxygen in order to make ATP, which is essentially the "energy" on which our bodies run. If there isn't adequate energy, then the neurons (the cells responsible for receiving sensory input from the outside world and for sending motor commands to our muscles) fail and many forms of neurological dysfunction and chronic health problems may follow.

Oxygen deprivation isn't only a reality for people who need to be "on oxygen" or are constantly hooked up to a machine. In fact, I see many, many patients who are lacking oxygen because they're anemic. An anemic person may have decreased blood circulation issues which equals decreased oxygen to the tissues of the body. Many of my patients have been anemic for years but no doctor has taken the time to explain to them what that means for their health so they don't understand the full implications of that diagnosis.

Our bodies must have an adequate supply of oxygen in order to heal, especially when it comes to chronic health problems. Oxygen plays a crucial role in helping us heal from chronic health issues because of something called "resting membrane potential of the nerve cells." When a nerve is asked to perform a task but it's lacking oxygen, it's similar to an empty soap dispenser. You can pump and pump but nothing is going to happen. On the contrary, when the dispenser is full, it may be so primed that soap is coming out without any pumping. In the same way, oxygen impacts the nervous system's ability to function because it's what "primes the pump" for the nerve cells and gives it the energy to do its job.

The nervous system is made up of individual cells called neurons, and to maintain the health of these neurons, oxygen is crucial. Healthy neurons and an optimally functioning nervous system are essential building blocks for structural integrity of the cells, fighting chronic health issues and healing the body. Let's take a moment to dive deeper into understanding neurons and their function in our bodies.

A neuron's job is to transmit communication from the brain to the body and from the body back to the brain. Neurons communicate in two ways: electronically (similar to the electrical system in your home) and chemically (called neurotransmitters). In order for neurons to optimize communication between the brain and the body (and vice versa), they need three things: oxygen, glucose, and stimulation. If any of one of those three elements are taken away, you get neurons that don't "fire" properly, and malfunctioning neurons may cause brain fog, attention, memory issues as well as numbness, tingling and pins and needles sensation in the body. If these neurons are interfered with, stunted, blunted or damaged in any way, the stage is set for an environment of dysfunction, which then may lead to a disease process.

To understand the disruptive effect of malfunctioning neurons, consider your home's internet connection. When the connection is interrupted or slowed, problems begin to appear. Your Netflix show appears grainy or your pictures don't download properly. Now think about your brain trying to communicate with all 75 trillion cells in your body. Imagine how easily things could go awry in that kind of system. So it is with our bodies and the complex wonder that is our neurological system. If the neurons that comprise our neurological system don't have an adequate supply of oxygen, the body can't heal itself properly because its main communication system is compromised.

There are a few ways to discover if you are oxygen deficient or not. To test a patient's oxygen levels at the clinic, I use a tool called a pulse oximeter. It's put on the tip of the finger and measures oxygen levels. Another way to test oxygen levels is by taking a person's blood pressure. If it's too low, it means the tissues of the body are not getting enough blood supply, and blood is what transports oxygen within the body. The third way to test oxygen levels is through blood work. I look at the total red blood cell count, and if that's too low, it's a sign of oxygen deficiency. These measurement tools are used to see how oxygen deficient someone may be and helps me determine how to treat them best. Signs of poor circulation are cold hands, cold feet, white fingernails (should be pink in color), and nail fungus. There's a saying in functional neurology, "cold hands, cold feet equals cold brain." Meaning, if you have poor circulation in your hands and feet, you probably have poor circulation in your brain as well.

RESULTS FROM OXYGEN

In order to understand how important oxygen is for healing chronic health problems, the main thing to grasp is that a person's oxygen level determines how much stimulation can be put into their nervous system before it "fails" (aka ceases to properly relay the stimulation). This system failure is known as "exceeding metabolic capacity" or

EMC. At that point, the nervous system can take no more stimulation and may react with a headache, dizziness, or equilibrium problems.

If you're suffering from anemia, the first thing you may experience is a lack of concentration, focus, and attention. This may eventually turn into memory loss and dementia, but if you catch it early enough, it may be reversed. Lack of oxygen may also cause your extremities to change color, your nails to turn white, or you may lack hair on your lower extremities.

When your body is deficient of oxygen, many internal systems begin to misfire and go awry. The signals traveling from the body to your brain travel at roughly 270 mph. If there's a lack of oxygen, those major neural pathways become compromised and can't convey those fast-moving signals. If your oxygen level is skewed at all, it can lead to numbness, tingling, sensations of pins and needles, and other strange symptoms that show the neurons are misfiring.

There are a few simple, at-home tests you can do to see if you are anemic, aka lacking oxygen and lack of circulation. Start by looking at your fingernails. Are they pink? (Pink is good.) Or are they white? (White is bad.) What color are your toes? Are they blue? (Blue is bad.) Or purple? (Purple very bad.) You can also check for "pitting edema." If you push your finger into your lower leg and it doesn't rebound quickly, you are likely anemic. Toe fungus is another clue that you're not getting enough oxygen to your extremities, or if you always have cold fingers and toes (or cold extremities in general) that's a sign of anemia and poor circulation.

Bloodwork is also a great way to tell if you're lacking oxygen. If you've had blood tests in the last six months, examine your results to see if your red blood cell (RBC) count is low. If it is, that's a clue. If your hemoglobin (HGB) is too low, you are anemic. If you have low hematocrit (HCT) that's also an indicator of anemia. Your blood is like the 18-wheeler that delivers oxygen to your body's tissues, so those numbers are solid indicators of whether you're getting adequate oxygen supply or not.

If you suspect you are anemic, increasing the supply of oxygen to your body may impact your overall health in many positive ways. First of all, you'll notice an increase in energy and endurance and your mental endurance will also improve. You may also notice a better ability to focus for long periods of time. Many patients tell me they start sleeping better, feel better and have more mental clarity. All of these positive results start to happen because the neurons have enough oxygen to fire properly.

YOUR FIRST STEP

There are many simple ways to increase your oxygen levels. At the clinic, I often have anemic patients do exercise with oxygen therapy. They put an oxygen supply mask over their face and then ride a stationary bike for 15 minutes, called Exercise With Oxygen Therapy (EWOT). This is a very powerful therapy for oxygenating the body as well as the brain, because not only is oxygen being pumped through the mask, but the body and brain naturally increase their ability to receive oxygen as well as improve circulation when performing EWOT.

A few other simple strategies to increase oxygen levels include walking for at least thirty minutes per day and doing deep breathing exercises. Deep breathing or "forced breathing" exercises actually help stimulate the frontal lobe areas of your brain. The key to forced breathing is a 1:2 ratio. Start with breathing in deeply for four seconds and out for eight seconds, if you can perform this task move up to six seconds in and twelve seconds out. Optimal performance would be eight seconds in and sixteen seconds out. For chronic health sufferers, eight in and sixteen out will be a challenge. These activities cause stimulation to the neurological pathways and inundate the body with oxygen. If you can't currently walk for thirty minutes, start by walking for five or six minutes per day. The most important thing is to stimulate the neurological system. Motion is life! Bicycling, either on a stationary bike or outdoors, is also excellent. Don't forget about swimming, it's low impact on your joints and very beneficial to your health. Take what you have at home and use it. It doesn't cost you anything to go outside and walk or do some forced breathing exercises.

When you go for your daily walk, swing your arms in an over exaggerated fashion. Non-linear complex movements (figure eight motions or writing your A,B,C's) will stimulate your cerebellum which in turn stimulates your brain. It's a win-win because it not only gets blood flowing to the extremity doing the non-linear movement, it also increases blood flow to the part of the cerebellum and brain which controls your extremities.

Now that we've covered the key health element of oxygen, let's look at the next key to improving chronic health problems.

6

KEY 2 – GLUCOSE

THE ROLE OF GLUCOSE

You may have heard the word "glucose" before, but what exactly is it and why is it so important to our health? Glucose is simply our blood sugar, and it's the "fuel" that drives our nervous system. It plays an essential role in healing chronic problems because it supplies our nervous system with the energy it needs to do its job. Of course, healing only happens when our glucose is in optimal range (85–99) and when our A1C is below 5.6. Both of these numbers are a part of routine bloodwork.

In the same way that a car needs the proper fuel for its engine to start and to drive down the road, your nervous system needs the right levels of glucose to function optimally. Not only is the type of fuel important, the amount of fuel is key as well. If you don't have enough glucose, your body can't create the energy it needs to function. (Anything below 85 is hypoglycemia.) Yet if there's too much glucose present in your body, you'll feel slow, sluggish, and tired after eating. (Anything above 99 is hyperglycemia.) An abundance of glucose can also have a severely damaging effect on the nervous system. The higher the number, the more damaging the effects to your nervous system, brain, blood vessels and organs resulting in problems such as kidney failure or blindness.

There are a few ways to measure the glucose levels of your body. The first and most common way is through a simple blood test. Based on your results, you can see if your glucose (aka blood sugar) levels are too high or too low. The most simple, inexpensive (free!) at-home "test" to evaluate your glucose levels is to pay attention to the way you feel before and after meals.

If your blood sugar is too low (a condition known as "hypoglycemia"), you will feel a lack of concentration and focus as well as irritability prior to eating. Have you ever heard the term "hangry?" After you eat and your body becomes inundated with glucose, you'll start to feel better. If your glucose levels are too low, you may also have a tendency to wake up at night, have trouble sleeping, and often skip breakfast.

If your glucose levels are too high (known as "hyperglycemia"), you'll likely feel sleepy and sluggish after eating, especially if your meal contains lots of carbohydrates. Too much blood sugar may also cause you to be constantly thirsty, have headaches, or have trouble concentrating.

When your glucose levels are properly balanced, you don't experience the "hangry" feelings, the "crash" after a meal, or the constant cravings for sugars and starches. The only thing that should happen after you eat is that you feel full. That's it.

RESULTS FROM GLUCOSE

Let's dive deeper into what happens when you have a deficiency of glucose. The first symptoms of low blood sugar are the loss of focus, concentration, and attention. Many hypoglycemic people experience psychiatric symptoms like depression and anxiety, or they feel dizzy and have frequent headaches. These symptoms happen because the neurological system is lacking the fuel it needs to function properly.

If glucose is the "fuel" that your nervous system needs to run on and the fuel gauge begins flashing "low," (there's that check engine light again) problems are going to surface. Essentially, your body's fuel source becomes so low that your neurons can't fire properly and begin losing function. Your car runs out of gas.

On the flip side, when there's an excess of glucose in the body, it's like taking sandpaper to the outside of an electrical cord. Inside the plastic sheath of the cord, there's a metal wire, which conducts electricity, just like our nervous system. If you take sandpaper to that coating and rub through the outer sheath, you can't put the protective sheath back on, leaving the bare wire exposed.

Too much glucose in the body has the same effect on the myelin sheath surrounding your nerve fibers. Myelin is an insulating layer that forms around nerves, including those in the brain and spinal cord. It is made up of protein and fatty substances, and it allows electrical impulses to transmit quickly and efficiently along the nerve cells. If that myelin coating is worn through, it can't be replaced as long as your glucose level is high. Once the nerve is exposed, the body's electrical system starts to malfunction because it lacks the protection it needs.

An excess of glucose can also cause balance problems, stability problems, coordination issues, and trouble with focus, attention, and concentration. Extreme cases of hyperglycemia can also cause kidney malfunction, blindness, or require the amputation of limbs. When there is too much glucose present in the bloodstream, things like insulin resistance start to appear, which is the precursor to diabetes. Interestingly enough, "Type 3" diabetes, a proposed term to describe the interlinked association between Type 1 and Type 2 diabetes and Alzheimer's disease, is also known as dementia and occurs when neurons in the brain become unable to respond to insulin, which is essential for basic tasks, including memory and learning.

Whether you are *hypo*glycemic (too little glucose) or *hyper*glycemic (too much glucose), the reality is that neither condition is ideal. Balanced, stable blood sugar levels are the goal, and when you get your glucose leveled out, everything begins to improve. You may even begin sleeping better because REM cycles are affected by both hyper and hypoglycemia. Your overall body function may improve, especially your liver, kidney, bladder and digestive health. How and why? Your organ system has to communicate with your brain and your brain has to communicate with your organs and it does this through the Vagus Nerve. With balanced blood sugar, you'll enjoy more energy and less mental and physical fatigue.

YOUR FIRST STEPS

When I see patients, I'm looking for an optimal fasting glucose level on their blood panel of anywhere from 85–99 and A1C below 5.6. This is different from the "medical normal" range which is 70–110. When I see a patient over 99, I consider them pre-diabetic because at this level, insulin resistance is already starting to destroy their nerve function, brain function, blood vessel function and organ function. When a person hits 126, they've officially entered into a disease process known as diabetes.

Anything below 85 is hypoglycemia meaning there's too little glucose in your blood for the neurological system to run at its peak level. If hypoglycemia gets to an advanced stage, it can actually cause you to pass out because there's such a severe lack of fuel that your neurons can't fire.

Your first step to balancing your blood sugar and stabilizing your glucose levels is to understand how and why you got to where you are today. Here's where I'm going to give you some tough love. Unless you are a Type 1 diabetic (which is an autoimmune disorder), this Type 2 diabetes is a self-inflicted condition. You did this to yourself. Ouch, I know that's hard to hear. The good news is that you can also undo it! This is where personal responsibility really comes into play.

To immediately begin stabilizing your glucose levels, I encourage you to start moving. Exercise burns off glucose, stimulates your nervous system, and increases your body's oxygen levels. Win, win, and win! Start with simple forms of movement like walking or bicycling, and then work up to more strenuous activities like swimming, workout classes, or weight lifting. Regardless of where you're at in your health journey, find a form of exercise that you enjoy and start doing it. Try to move your body every day. Again, motion is life! If you rest, you rust.

The second key to stabilizing your blood sugar is found in the kitchen. It's all about what you put in your mouth. What you put *in* your mouth is just as important as the way you move your body. Start tracking your food using a phone app like MyFitnessPal to find out how many grams of carbs and sugar you're consuming each day. You don't have to track your food forever, but committing to it for 60–90 days is one of the best tools to teach you how to eat properly. Most people are shocked when they see their initial numbers. Get rid of the bread, cake, and cookies. Eat less carbs and consume more healthy proteins and fats (baked chicken, fish, bison). Portion sizes are also crucial. Measure out your meals carefully and skip on seconds.

Glucose is essential for solving chronic health problems because it's the fuel that our neurological system needs to do its job. However, having too much or too little glucose can cause serious health issues and even create serious disease processes like diabetes. Doing these simple things can help you conquer your goal of achieving long-term health through stable glucose levels. Now that we've talked about glucose, let's move on to the next key to solving chronic health problems—stimulation.

7

KEY 3 – STIMULATION

THE ROLE OF STIMULATION

The definition of neurostimulation is "the activation of a nerve through an external source." Touch, for example, is a kind of stimulation as well as walking, cycling or swimming. Seeing something new is a form of stimulation. Hearing your friend speak is a form of stimulation. Picking up a 5lb weight and doing a bicep curl is a type of stimulation. When it comes to the neurological system, neural pathways need stimulation in order to be healthy. These pathways are designed to send information and signals (both electrically and chemically) from the body to the brain and the brain to the body, and don't forget your organ system is part of your body. Think of the neurological system like a muscle. If it's stimulated, it grows and gets stronger. If it's not stimulated, it begins to atrophy just like a muscle that isn't used enough.

It's crucial to understand the role that stimulation plays in solving chronic health problems because this is an area of health that's so often overlooked. Stimulation is required to stabilize neurological function. When a system is under-stimulated, it begins to atrophy and so does the area of the brain that controls that body part. To solve this problem, I use targeted, specific types of stimulation to "fire" those pathways. This activation creates more neuro-plasticity and increases the function of that area of the neurological systems. Neuro-plasticity (also known as "brain plasticity") is the ability of the brain and nervous system to modify its connections or rewire itself. Stimulating certain areas of the nervous system in specific ways makes the brain fire better which can solve problems in the body.

Different parts of the body are connected to different parts of the brain. For instance, if you are having problems with smell, taste, memory, or vision, all of those senses fire through your temporal lobe which means that part of your brain needs a certain kind of stimulation to get it working again. The reason we have to understand stimulation is because we need to find out what part of the brain is malfunctioning and figure out which systems we need to stimulate to bring that part of the brain back online.

For example, if a patient breaks their arm, their arm is going to atrophy within two weeks. They can eat broccoli and cauliflower and asparagus every day, five times per day, but if they don't stimulate the arm muscles, they're going to get smaller. The only way to make this muscle grow is to stimulate it. Specifically, a person with a broken arm, once the arm is out of the cast, needs the stimulation of bicep curls and tricep extensions to bring it and the part of their brain that controls their arm back to full working capacity. Doing calf raises, even though it's a form of stimulation, wouldn't help heal their arm because it's the wrong kind of stimulation. This method is known as "receptor-based activation," and it uses movement and stimulation to activate the brain.

Certain parts of the brain perform certain functions and control specific parts of the body. When we experience problems in our body, it's often because certain parts of the brain are not functioning as they should. Stimulating different parts of the brain in specific ways makes it "fire" or signal better which in turn solves problems in the body, and some of the stories that have come from treating patients through receptor-based activation have been nothing short of amazing.

A few years ago, a man came into the clinic and was having major balance issues. In fact, his balance was so poor that the only way he could move down the hallway was by putting his forearms against the wall and shuffling his feet side to side. He'd been to every kind of doctor and undergone many different forms of treatment, yet nothing had helped him walk normally. After I talked with him and did a neurological examination, it became clear that he needed receptor-based activation in his front core muscle group. I told him to do bicep curls for twenty seconds, and immediately after he did, he walked normally without any assistance. Why did this treatment work so fast? Because stimulating the correct area of the brain helped it become balanced, and it functioned more optimally because of it. Correct neurological stimulation is an amazing modality.

RESULTS OF STIMULATION

What actually happens when the body has a deficiency of stimulation? To understand the inner workings of the human brain, we first need to wrap our minds around the massive amount of energy that it requires to operate. The brain weighs about three pounds, and it is very metabolically demanding, consuming 25–30% of our overall oxygen and glucose intake. Consider that for a moment. Almost one third of the oxygen and glucose brought into our bodies is used by the brain alone. It is by far the most energy demanding organ, and because of that, the brain requires a constant supply of oxygen and glucose.

If the brain has the right amounts of oxygen and glucose, the final key that it needs to maintain optimal health is—you guessed it—proper neurological stimulation. It's the final piece of the Big Three (oxygen, glucose, stimulation) for maintaining a healthy, vibrant neurological system. If there's a lack of stimulation, the neurons will begin to break down and no longer produce the electrical and chemical activation to maintain neuronal health, which in turn causes the neurological pathways to atrophy. The atrophy of the pathways also causes atrophy in the brain. If you don't use it you lose it. In order for the neurological system to be healthy, it must be stimulated. If you want your arms to be strong, you have to do push-ups. If you don't, you'll have skinny, weak arms. If you don't stimulate your brain and neurological pathways, they break down as well, and the first signs of loss of brain health is brain fog, and the loss of focus, attention and concentration.

If the idea of your brain atrophying and your neurological pathways malfunctioning doesn't sound pleasant, I have good news for you. There may be a solution to your problem! You can increase the level of neurological stimulation and improve your health in a multitude of ways. When you increase stimulation in your daily life, you may experience an increased memory capacity, better vision, a clearer memory, a better sense of taste and smell, and more appreciation for touch. With all of these exciting benefits to gain, let's dig into strategies for self-testing and improving stimulation in your daily life.

YOUR FIRST STEPS – EVALUATION AND STIMULATION

There are several simple ways to test the health of your neurological pathways. The first indicator of a healthy brain is your ability to learn new information, to stay focused, and to concentrate on the topic at hand. When is the last time you learned something for the first time? The only long-term way to maintain the health of your brain is to stimulate it by trying new things, tasting new foods, smelling new smells, seeing new sights, and going to new places. Pay attention to how mentally "rigid" you are towards new ideas or plans. People who are inflexible and have a "my way or the highway" mentality often have very unhealthy brains.

When I examine the health of a patient's brain, there are four main areas of the brain that I consider: the temporal lobe, the parietal lobe, the frontal lobe, and the prefrontal lobe (or prefrontal cortex). The temporal lobe controls taste, smell, memory, and vision. The parietal lobe is in charge of body sensation and vision. The frontal lobe controls voluntary movement, and the prefrontal cortex handles focus, attention, concentration, memory, impulse control, and motivation. The deficiency of stimulation also determines which part of the brain is malfunctioning, and this is all determined through neurological testing. I have many tests that I do at my clinic, but there are also easy, at-home testing strategies for each lobe of the brain.

Temporal lobe self-test: Ask yourself these questions: "Can I taste and smell things as I did before? Have my senses increased, decreased or stayed the same? (If they've decreased, that indicates a lack of stimulation in the temporal lobe). How's my memory? Am I as "sharp" as ever or has my memory declined?"

Parietal lobe self-test: One simple test is called the Digit Span Test. Here's how you perform it. You need a partner. Close your eyes and have your partner touch two of your toes on one foot. Can you identify how many toes are between the toes your partner is touching? Now repeat on the other foot and well as your fingers on both hands. If this neurological system is damaged, you will not be able to identify what your partner is doing.

Frontal lobe self-test: Do I move as well now as I did in the past or has my movement slowed? How is my memory compared to years past? Am I becoming more irritated over trivial things? Am I becoming more inflexible? The biggest problem with frontal lobe issues is that you don't see the change but everyone around you does. It's strange but with frontal lobe demise, we can't see it in ourselves but everyone else can see our deficiencies.

Prefrontal cortex self-test: A healthy prefrontal cortex is essential for planning, and execution of complex issues such as behavior, speech, and logical reasoning, as well as impulse control, motivation, understanding the consequences of your actions, and short term memory. If you've noticed you're not following through with what you've started, planning poorly, having short term memory as well as lacking impulse control, then your prefrontal cortex may need some rehab.

CEREBELLUM:

Stability test (do this with caution): Put your feet together (side-by-side), close your eyes, and hold that position for 15 seconds. Next, put your right foot in front of the left, close your eyes and hold for 15 seconds. Lastly, put your left foot in front of your right foot, close your eyes, and hold for 15 seconds.

Flex test (do this with caution): Stand on one leg with the other leg lifted and flexed at 90 degrees, then hold that position for 15 seconds. Repeat on the other side.

These cerebellar tests are very important for stability and balance. Count out loud and see how long you can maintain your balance and stability. A health cerebellum will allow for the full fifteen seconds for each test.

These simple at-home tests can give you an idea of how your neurological pathways are currently firing, and if you performed the tests and didn't like the results, don't fear. Here are some exercises you can do to stimulate those pathways and "fire" your brain back up.

Non-linear complex movements: You can actually do these exercises while you're sitting down at the table or relaxing on your couch. Start by sitting down or standing up, then do a figure eight in the air with your arm or "write" the name of your city and state in the air, write your ABCs, your name, etc. Try writing your name in the air with your hand and leg at the same time. This fires your cerebellum, frontal lobe and the parietal lobe at that same time. Pair this with deep breathing and you're really stimulating your brain and giving it plenty of oxygen to increase the level of stimulation your neurological system can take.

Deep breathing exercises: As stated before deep breathing or forced breathing stimulates frontal lobe function. Start slowly and build up and remember the 1:2 ratio. Breathe in four seconds and out eight seconds. Once you can perform 4:8 move up to 6:12, six seconds in and twelve seconds out. Next step is 8:16, eight seconds in and sixteen seconds out. It won't be easy getting to 8:16 but remember, things worth having are hardly ever easy.

8

KEY 4 – AUTOIMMUNE DISORDERS

THE ROLE OF AUTOIMMUNE (AI) DISORDERS

Before we dig into autoimmune disorders and their profound impact on your health, let's first look at the driver of autoimmunity which is your immune system. So what is an immune system, exactly, and why is it important to your body? Your immune system is basically your built-in SEAL Team 6. It's your body's special defense mechanism against all of the antigens of the world. An antigen is any substance that sparks your immune system to produce antibodies such as chemicals, bacteria, cancer cells, viruses, or pollen. Your immune system recognizes that these antigens are not meant to be inside of you and then activates to fight off and kill the offender. When you develop an autoimmune condition, your immune system begins attacking your own tissues because it thinks your tissue is the antigen. Essentially, an autoimmune condition is "friendly fire" within your body.

Autoimmune (AI) conditions can be devastating to patients suffering with chronic health problems because AI can not only exacerbate existing chronic problems, but AI by itself is the health problem. The autoimmune condition acts like the Tasmanian devil inside your body, wreaking havoc and causing damage. Once an autoimmune condition begins destroying things, it can cause a whole host of other seemingly unrelated issues.

One of the biggest drivers of autoimmune conditions that I see in my clinic is a sensitivity to gluten. Gluten is a protein found in wheat and is in manufactured cereal, grains, pasta, bread and flour, just to name a few products. It is the substance that makes bread dough elastic and stretchy, and it is devastating to the human brain. Gluten is one of the most destructive proteins found on the planet today, and no, it's not the same wheat that our ancestors consumed centuries ago. It's a commercialized, hybridized version that our body can no longer recognize or break down. As a result, undigested gluten proteins work their way into the bloodstream and spark an immune response. Since gluten's amino acid profile closely resembles the amino acid profile of the human thyroid gland and cerebellum tissue, this immune response quickly turns into an autoimmune response that attacks those parts of your body.

Every single human needs to test their tolerance for gluten, and the test I recommend is panel A2 from www.Enterolab.com. You can order this test directly from the company. Another test is Cyrex Array 3, but a doctor has to order this test. This is a genetic test which identifies whether or not you carry the gluten sensitivity gene and if it has been turned on. It also tells you whether or not you have the Celiac gene. I can't stress enough how important it is for everyone to become educated on gluten intolerance and their body's reaction to wheat and other cereal grains.

RESULTS FROM AUTOIMMUNE DISORDERS

When your body is battling an autoimmune disorder, it could appear as a multitude of other, seemingly unrelated chronic health problems. Ataxia, which is an unstable posture or irregular gait, is commonly linked to autoimmune disease. Thyroid problems like Hashimoto's Disease can be rooted in autoimmune conditions. Recent research has suggested approximately 90% of people who have thyroid issues also have an autoimmune disorder. Fibromyalgia is a chronic disorder characterized by widespread musculoskeletal pain, fatigue, and tenderness in localized areas and is often rooted in autoimmune problems. Cerebellum issues like blurred vision, balance problems, and uncoordinated movements with your hands and feet are all signals that you may be dealing with an autoimmune condition.

Other signs of autoimmune disease are general cognitive decline like a lack of focus, attention and concentration. Dementia, forgetting things like names, numbers, and dates, is a concerning signal of an autoimmune condition. Psychological disorders like panic, anxiety, depression, and irrational fear are often rooted in autoimmune causes as well. Migraine headaches, multiple sclerosis, ALS (often called Lou Gehrig's disease), stiffness in movements, tremors, and restless leg syndrome are all chronic conditions that are closely linked to autoimmune roots with the majority of these reactions being triggered by the gluten found in modern wheat.

Many people mistakenly think that only people diagnosed with Celiac disease are intolerant to gluten, however the truth is that only about 30% of people who have Celiac disease have gut-related issues. The other 70% have a myriad of other problems. Celiac disease destroys the microvilli, the tiny hair-like projections within the small intestine that increase nutrient absorption. These projections increase the surface area of the small intestine allowing more area for nutrients to be absorbed. Celiac destroys these microvilli to the point that they can't absorb nutrients. When they are damaged, it kicks off a host of other disease processes that can turn into full-blown autoimmune conditions.

YOUR FIRST STEP

When the gut becomes inflamed and damaged, harmful proteins like gluten cross the blood-brain barrier and "dock" in the part of your brain where your opioid receptors live. This means people who regularly eat breads, cakes, cookies, brownies, and other foods containing wheat flour are truly addicted to these foods. When they eat them, their brain reacts very similarly to someone consuming opioids. What's your reaction as you've read my encouragement to ditch wheat and gluten? Did you say, "No way! I can't live without my (fill in the blank)." If those thoughts crossed your mind, there's a good chance you're addicted to gluten.

I can't encourage you strongly enough—get gluten out of your life. The side effects are absolutely devastating. If you want to learn more about the bad effects of gluten, I highly recommend the book Grain Brain by David Perlmutter, MD. It goes into much more detail on the effects that modern gluten has on the human brain.

If you suspect that you have a lurking autoimmune condition, don't lose hope. It may be possible to slow down the damage, and in some cases even reverse it IF caught early enough. Here comes "tough love part two." The most important point for you to remember is this: improving the lives of patients suffering with chronic health problems begins with my patients taking personal responsibility. Most autoimmune conditions are triggered by lifestyle choices which means that they can also be improved upon through major lifestyle changes. These kinds of changes can be challenging to make, but what is your health worth to you? That's the question you need to answer when you look in the mirror, "Am I worth it?" Only you can answer that question.

The first step to identifying an autoimmune condition is to order the www.EnteroLab.com panel A2 test. If I was a betting kind of guy, I would wager that you do have the gluten sensitivity gene. If you have a gluten sensitivity problem, it's crucial that you avoid gluten at all costs and get on an autoimmune paleo diet. You also need to start the Freedom Metabolic Restore Program.

Will you make mistakes? Absolutely! Anyone taking on a major lifestyle change will slip up and fall off "the bandwagon" as we say, but don't let those mistakes keep you from getting back on the program. Keep heading in the right direction and you will begin to see improvement.

A great first step in the right direction is to deep clean your home of all products containing gluten. This includes cooking devices like toasters that have touched your bread, English muffins, etc. Throw away all wheat flours, breads, cookies, baking mixes, and more. With a wheat and gluten sensitivity, you're either all in or you're out. You can't be 95% in, you have to be 100% committed because once you consume gluten, it takes months for it to completely leave your system.

Take heart. There is hope. You can get rid of all the negative side effects of gluten while still enjoying your life. However, it takes time and commitment for these changes to become part of your new lifestyle. If you're willing to put in the work, I can almost guarantee you'll see a significant improvement in your health. Now that we've covered autoimmune disorders, let's move to the next key to solving chronic health problems.

9

KEY 5 – INFLAMMATION

THE ROLE OF INFLAMMATION

Inflammation—this is a term we hear often, but do we really know what it is, why it happens, and why we often have too much of it? Let's start by discussing what inflammation is supposed to do. In its proper context, inflammation is actually a good thing because it acts as a signaling agent to tell the body to start repairing, restoring, and regenerating itself. This regeneration is kicked off by the formation of new blood vessels. Nothing can heal until new blood vessels are created (called angiogenesis), and in this regard, inflammation is a positive thing.

Inflammation comes to the rescue when you experience an acute injury like a twisted ankle, a dislocated shoulder, or a badly banged shin. In that context, inflammation is a localized physical condition that causes the body to become swollen, red, and hot to the touch. This is when inflammation signals to the rest of the body to begin the healing process. The trouble begins when inflammation gets out of hand and out of homeostasis.

Homeostasis is the body's ability to maintain a relatively stable internal state that persists despite changes in the world outside. When there isn't homeostasis, disease processes can begin to develop. As with many parts of our health, inflammation causes problems when it goes rogue and there is too much of it.

Inflammation becomes a major issue when it's continually present in the body. This can happen for a variety of reasons. In this scenario, inflammation in the body is like fire inside of a house. It's totally destructive and stands in the way of optimizing chronic issues. Some of the most common signs of chronic inflammation are actually more psychological than physical. Brain fog, depression, anxiety, irritability, and fatigue are all signs of chronic inflammation of the brain. When chronic inflammation exists in the brain, that dreaded brain fog is almost always the first symptom to appear. Sometimes I compare it to feeling like the "walking dead" or like you're living in zombie land. You have a hard time focusing, concentrating, and staying hooked on one task for an extended period of time.

Inflammation plays a distinct and important role in healing chronic disease because it's something we must eliminate before we can begin untangling the web of dysfunction and healing the root issue. If a house was on fire, would you start rebuilding it before the fire was completely put out? No, that would be ridiculous. In the same way, we have to eradicate the chronic inflammation before we can begin rebuilding the body. If there's chronic inflammation present, it's going to accelerate the degeneration in your brain, joints, nervous system, and circulatory system much more quickly. If you're dealing with any kind of inflammation anywhere, you have to zap it before you can start to heal.

Bloodwork is the most accurate way to measure the level of inflammation present in the body. The A1C markers on a blood panel can be used to measure inflammation. The CRP (c-reactive protein) and the homocysteine markers also indicate inflammation levels. Everyone has some level of inflammation present in their system at all times, but these tests are used to see if it is out of control or not. This information is used to make a plan for reducing the level of chronic inflammation in your system.

RESULTS OF INFLAMMATION

So what causes this kind of chronic inflammation? The factors can be both psychological and physical. Psychological things like being overworked, excessively difficult workouts, unhealthy relationships, a stressful job, and not having enough "me time" can all contribute to chronic inflammation of the brain.

Physical causes of chronic inflammation can be obvious things like slipping and falling, a car wreck (even if it was several years ago), whiplash, repetitive injuries or motions, falling out of a tree, falling off a ladder, and more. Chronic inflammation from these kinds of traumatic injuries can stay with you many years, even after the more obvious symptoms disappear.

A glucose imbalance (see Chapter 6), anemia, leaky gut syndrome, leaky brain syndrome, and food sensitivities can cause out-of-control inflammation in the body. When these things occur, the body releases cortisol to combat the stress of the inflammatory process. Cortisol is a stress-related hormone that is meant to help control blood sugar levels, regulate metabolism, help reduce inflammation, and assist with memory formulation. However, when the body signals cortisol to be released over and over again, the negative effects begin to spiral out of control. If there's too much cortisol in your system, it can affect the quality of your sleep. It also directly attacks the hippocampus, the region of the brain that is associated primarily with memory.

Decreasing the level of inflammation in your system will positively affect your health in many, many ways. First of all, it will save your brain. That sounds extreme, but it's true. The brain is very sensitive to inflammation, and by decreasing the level of inflammation in the brain, you're going to avoid many memory, focus and concentration, and anxiety driven problems. When you put out the "fire in the house," your focus, attention, and brain fog issues should significantly decrease. You should have an increased ability to think more clearly and experience a clarity of mind and senses that you haven't noticed for quite a while. As you work to decrease the inflammation in your body, your pain syndromes should start to decrease. Your joint pain may slow down or be completely eliminated, and you may even notice your balance improving.

If your inflammation levels are out of control, the first thing to do is look at is your diet. You can take all the anti-inflammatory products in the world, but you can't out-supplement a poor diet. You can't out-medicate it either. Making the necessary dietary changes (most commonly, eliminating gluten, sugar, and casein, the protein found in milk) is a major first step to reducing inflammation and healing chronic disease.

YOUR FIRST STEPS

So what can you do, starting today, to begin decreasing the inflammation level in your body? What a great question! The exciting thing is that there is a lot you can do to help put out the fire and set the stage for true healing. First let's talk about psychological and physiological things you can do to reduce one of the biggest drivers of inflammation, which is stress.

If you notice stress playing a major inflammatory role in your life, start incorporating important mental health practices like regular deep tissue massage and "unplugging" from technology on a regular basis. No one is going to care more about your brain and bodily health than you, and *you* need to make these things a major priority in your life. All of these things are an investment in your long-term health. Make a commitment to disconnect from technology for one day per week. Schedule a ninety minute massage once per month. Listen to soothing music. Go to a happy, funny movie and laugh for a whole hour straight. Listen to soothing nature sounds. Eliminate the bad and unnecessarily stressful relationships from your life. If you're in a bad relationship, discontinue it or take the hard but necessary steps to improve it. All of these small changes add up to a major effect. It's like a snowball that's rolling down a hill. At first, the changes seem minor, but as you pick up speed, the momentum becomes undeniable.

As far as physical changes that can help decrease inflammation, there are a lot of them. First of all, stop eating gluten, casein, and sugar. These substances do nothing but cause inflammation and wreak havoc on your gut-brain health. Stop eating processed foods that are filled with inflammatory oils and Trans Fats. Examples of trans fats include, but are not limited to, store bought cakes, cookies and pies, shortening, microwave popcorn, frozen pizza, fried foods, doughnuts, non-dairy creamer, and margarine. No wonder you're having headaches, brain fog and your feet are tingling and numb. In addition to dietary changes, you can incorporate other physical things like using an inversion table or adding nutritional supplements into your daily routine.

I think everyone should be taking an omega-3 fish oil supplement, and lots of it. The bare minimum daily required amount is 500mg but you can take up to 5000mg with zero negative side effects. Take the best kind you can afford. If you've had a bad experience with Omega-3 supplements in the past, it may be because you took a poor quality supplement. Up your intake of foods high in antioxidants, aka super foods. This includes things like purple, red or blue grapes (make sure they have seeds in them and eat the seeds as well), blueberries, raspberries, raw almonds, walnuts, pecans, kale, spinach (see, Popeye was right), broccoli, sweet potatoes, green or black tea, beans, and fish. These substances help rid the body of free radicals caused by inflammation. Drink real, home-brewed green tea. I recommend buying through Tea Market Spice in Seattle, Washington (phone number 800-735-7198.) My favorite varieties are the Japanese green tea (#3577) and the China mountain green tea (#5577).

When you begin to incorporate these lifestyle changes into your daily routine, you will be amazed at the way your body and brain feel.

Eliminating inflammation in your body is a fantastic step toward healing chronic health problems and regaining your health and vibrancy. Now that we've talked about inflammation, let's move onto the next key – environmental toxins.

10

KEY 6 – NEUROTOXINS

THE ROLE OF NEUROTOXINS

A neurotoxin is something you ingest into your body that has a direct link to brain and neurological destruction. The word "neurotoxin" may spark images of strange green substances bubbling in chemistry class, but the reality is that neurotoxins are hiding in some of the most ingested substances on earth. In fact, you probably have many of these substances in your kitchen right now, and understanding the role these toxins play in either starting or continuing chronic health problems is crucial. As your body digests and breaks down a neurotoxic substance, it may either trigger an autoimmune attack or kick off some kind of destructive brain and/or body disease process.

Here's a list of the most common neurotoxins that the majority of Americans consume every day:

- Wheat, particularly the gluten (the protein found in wheat), is the most destructive protein you can ever put in your body therefore it is classified as a neurotoxin. Again, I recommend the book Grain Brain by David Perlmutter, MD.

- Common table sugar is also a neurotoxin. As your body breaks it down, your blood sugar becomes spiked, which triggers a release of insulin which in turn produces a destructive inflammatory response.
- High fructose corn syrup is highly inflammatory. Most commonly used as a sweetener in sodas and other sweet drinks, high fructose corn syrup triggers a similar inflammatory response as table sugar. Because of this, I highly suggest you stop drinking sodas immediately.
- Artificial sweeteners are very toxic to the brain. Though they seem innocent because they don't contain sugar, they harm the brain in a different way. They contain a substance that causes our bodies' glutamate, an excitatory neurotransmitter, to over react to the product. It's similar to slamming the gas pedal of your car to the floor while it's in park and over-revving the engine to the point of blowing it up. These artificial sweeteners do the same thing to your glutamate neurotransmitters and essentially blow their doors off. To avoid artificial sweeteners, stop drinking diet soda as well as other diet beverages. For more information on the topic, I recommend you read *Excitotoxins: The Taste That Kills* by Russell Blaylock, MD.
- Monosodium Glutamate (MSG) is another substance that has a similar effect on your sensory neurotransmitters as the artificial sweeteners. This substance over-excites those receptors to the point of malfunction and degeneration which then leads to negative psychological side effects like brain fog, depression, and anxiety. To avoid MSG, steer clear of processed foods like flavored tortilla chips, ranch dressing mixes, some soy sauces and prepackaged Asian foods, and other highly processed items.
- Trans fats are hydrogenated oils that are highly inflammatory to the body. Anything that is inflammatory over a long period of time is going to destroy your brain function so avoiding anything that contains trans fats is crucial.

- Drinking bottled water from the commonly sold plastic disposable bottles has proven to be a source of neurotoxic material. Avoiding the consumption of and exposure to these plastic products greatly reduces the toxic load on your body's detoxification systems.
- There are a few more common neurotoxic culprits like heavy metals—lead, mercury, and formaldehyde, and these toxic substances are found in some unsuspecting places. Recent medical studies have shown that lead poisoning may be generational. The results showed that if a parent got lead poisoning, it took roughly 4 generations to get it out of their offspring's system. Mercury (aka thimerosal) is found in vaccines, as well as aluminum, which is in most underarm deodorants.

RESULTS FROM NEUROTOXINS

Understanding the realities and effects of neurotoxins plays an important role in helping people optimize their chronic issues. Since these neurotoxins damage the brain, the body's most important healing organ, it only stands to reason that removing substances which hurt the brain will accelerate healing. When there's a large amount of neurotoxins present in your body, it accelerates the degeneration of your joints, causes focus and concentration issues, can increase fear and anxiety, activate autoimmune disorders and destroy body tissue. Many chronic diseases, movement disorders, fibromyalgia, burning and numbness, tingling and coordination problems can be linked to an overload of neurotoxins.

These negative effects are often overlooked because most people, even traditional doctors, don't understand the link between inflammation of the brain and one's ability to improve their chronic condition. A brain and body detox as well as an elimination diet are very useful tools for changing your body's chemistry and your lifestyle so you can kick these nasty toxins to the curb.

Decreasing your consumption of neurotoxins will also yield some very nice lifestyle benefits like better sleep (the more cortisol you have, the less melatonin you release therefore making it harder to fall asleep and stay asleep), decreased pain and discomfort, better bowel movements, improved sexual function, better concentration and focus, and greater stability and balance.

YOUR FIRST STEPS

Your first step is to remember that you have the power to stop eating, drinking, and surrounding yourself with foods and substances that are neurotoxic to your brain. Stop eating the processed foods and quit drinking sodas, both traditional and diet. Stop buying plastic water bottles and instead invest in a glass water bottle that you refill at home with reverse osmosis water. If you have coffee, make sure you drink only organic coffee. Flavor your water with lemon or lime juice instead of ingesting traditional soda drinks or artificial sweeteners. There are many, many ways to enjoy the things you love like a great cup of coffee or a refreshing beverage without sacrificing your health.

The bottom line is to eliminate the neurotoxins listed above. Are there other toxins out there besides the ones I talked about in this book? Absolutely. There are herbicides, pesticides, environmental toxins, and more, but your exposure to those are mostly out of your control. Instead of focusing on what we can't control, let's focus on what we can control. You get to control everything you put in your mouth and on your body. Those daily choices are either healing you or slowly killing you, and you get to decide which direction you choose.

11

KEY 7 – THE BRAIN-GUT CONNECTION

THE ROLE OF GUT HEALTH

What is your "gut?" What does it have to do with healing chronic disease and untangling the web of dysfunction? Why does the condition of your gut matter so much for your overall health picture? How is gut health connected to the well-being of your brain? We're going to answer all of these important questions and more in this chapter.

For starters, your "gut" is not referring to the roundness we get around our midsection when we eat too many Christmas cookies. Instead, the term "gut health" refers to the physical state and physiologic function of the many parts of the gastrointestinal tract, also called the Enteric Nervous System. At one time, our digestive system was considered a relatively "simple" body system, but as our understanding of the gut and its many functions has grown, it's proven to be anything but simple. The gut not only consists of many different organs which work together to withdraw nutrition from our food, it also is home to trillions of microorganisms which live in our intestines. These microorganisms are a mixture of beneficial and non-beneficial bacteria, and in a healthy, optimally functioning gut, the "good bugs" far outnumber the "bad bugs." What's even more amazing is that these microorganisms are an essential part of your immune system, and over 70% of your immune system is found in your gut. The health and wellness of these microorganisms greatly depends on the foods we eat, the stress we endure, the medications we take, and the environment we live in.

In recent years, more attention has been paid to the importance of gut health and the way an unhealthy gut contributes to the web of dysfunction. The gut is so crucial to our overall wellness for more reasons than digesting food and extracting nutrients. Your gut (Enteric Nervous System) is connected to your brain via the Vagus Nerve, and in fact, they're so connected that we should almost view them as one system. If one is damaged, dysfunction in the other is sure to follow.

The link between the gut and the brain is known as the "gut/brain axis." The two are so interconnected that they're basically one, ultra complex system. The human gut (Enteric Nervous System) is lined with more than 500 million nerve cells so it's practically a brain unto itself. To give you an example, the human spinal cord has approximately 100 million nerve cells. Because the Gut/Brain axis is so interconnected, in order to heal one, you have to also heal the other. The neuro-metabolic web of dysfunction really starts to untangle when you solve the problems with your Gut/Brain Axis.

There are two main ways that the brain and the gut communicate with one another, and either of these modes of communication can be disrupted by trauma or inflammation. The first way the brain and gut communicate is through the Vagus nerve, a large "super highway" kind of nerve that extends from the brain stem to part of the colon. It also happens to be the longest cranial nerve in the body.

The second way the gut and the brain communicate is through the Central Autonomic Network which is also known as the "C.A.N." This complex network can be compromised by trauma as well as physiological or psychological issues. Any kind of damage to either the function of the Vagus nerve or the C.A.N. may spark leaky gut syndrome in your body. In fact, research suggests that within 6–12 hours after trauma happens to the brain (concussion, whiplash injury), you will have a leaky gut.

Your digestive system plays a key role in protecting your body from harmful substances. The walls of the intestines act as barriers, kind of like screen doors in our home, controlling what enters the bloodstream to be transported to your organs. If that screen is compromised, the barrier is breached and bugs get into the house. We have these kinds of protective barriers in our brain and gut and when they're damaged, trouble occurs. The inflammatory cascade starts here.

Small gaps in the intestinal wall called "tight junctions" allow water and nutrients to pass through, while blocking the passage of harmful substances. When these tight junctions are damaged to the point that they open up and no longer prevent harmful substances from passing into the bloodstream, it is known as "leaky gut syndrome." Leaky gut can be summarized in two words—intestinal permeability. When the gut is "leaky" and bacteria and other antigens enter the bloodstream, it can cause widespread inflammation and potentially trigger a reaction from the immune system. Those harmful substances are supposed to simply pass through the digestive tract, and when they breach that barrier and get into your bloodstream, they wreak all kinds of havoc.

Gluten sensitivity as well as an overload of neurotoxins can also cause damage and result in a leaky gut. The reason that gut health is so crucial is because if your gut isn't healthy and doing its job, it affects every other system in the body. To solve the riddle of chronic health issues and begin to untangle the neuro-metabolic web of dysfunction, we have to address brain function and gut function. That's why gut health is one of my seven keys to healing chronic health issues.

Gut health plays a distinct role in fostering true health and healing chronic disease because of the key role it plays in your immune system. As I mentioned earlier, about 70% of your immune system is found in your gut. To foster true health, you also need homeostasis between your sympathetic and parasympathetic nervous systems. Your Vagus nerve, the nerve that runs from the brainstem all the way to the colon, is what controls all of these functions.

To measure your gut health, there are several good blood work tests that show whether your gut is functioning correctly or not. The www.EnteroLab.com panel A2 test indicates if the gut is functioning properly. If you have an immune response to milk, wheat, soy or eggs, you likely have a leaky gut. If you have a leaky gut, you have a leaky brain.

RESULTS FROM GUT HEALTH

When you have poor gut health, there are a whole host of problems that could be showing up in your life. Some of the physical maladies you may be experiencing include GERD (gastroesophageal reflux disease), Crohn's disease, irritable bowel syndrome, SIBO (small intestinal bacterial overgrowth), and gastric reflux. These common disease processes all find their roots in having a leaky gut.

Many psychological issues like brain fog, lack of focus and attention, depression, anxiety, and overwhelming fear can develop as a result of leaky gut because when the gut is not healthy, neither is the brain. As I said before, you cannot have a healthy brain unless you have a healthy gut. If you have damage to the brain or you're feeding your gut bad stuff, those barriers are compromised and it kicks off a wave of inflammation and autoimmune disorders.

YOUR FIRST STEPS

So what can you do, starting today, to increase your gut health?

1) Eliminate the seven most common neurotoxins (see chapter 10). If you damage your brain, you damage your gut and vice versa.

2) Complete the Freedom Metabolic Restore Program. Detoxifying your body and supporting your gut and brain health will kick start your path to healing and help you begin to untangle the web of dysfunction.
3) Do the nerve stimulation exercises below 3–4 times per week. Since the Vagus nerve is the main super highway which allows the gut and brain to communicate, stimulating the Vagus nerve regularly is a fantastic way to promote optimal gut health.

I also suggest some extremely high quality nutritional supplements. The supplements listed below are NOT FDA approved to treat and disease or cure any aliment, and is NOT to take the place of any medication your doctor may have prescribed.

i. *Apex Energetics – ClearVite-PSF (K-84) Part 1 of 3 of our Freedom Metabolic Restore Program. Helps support liver detoxification reactions, the biliary system, and sugar metabolism.*
ii. *Apex Energetics – RepairVite (K-60) Part 2 of 3 of our Freedom Metabolic Restore Program. Intended to support the intestinal tract and intestinal lining.*
iii. *Apex Energetics – Strengtia Probiotics (K-61) Part 3 of 3 of our Freedom Metabolic Restore Program. Designed to fortify the intestinal microbial environment with targeted probiotics.*
iv. *Apex Energetics – Ultra-D Complex (K-35) intended to support the brain and the immune system.*
v. *Apex Energetics – Protoglysen (K-28) and Glysen (K-1) Both are designed to support sugar metabolism and help buffer glycemic response.*
vi. *Apex Energetics – NeurO2 (K-45) uniquely designed and mechanistically balanced to support the cerebral microvascular for healthy blood flow to the brain.*
vii. *Apex Energetics – Neuro-Flam (K-46) is a phenol-flavonoid complex designed to specifically target brain health as it relates to microglial activity in the brain-immune system.*

viii. *Apex Energetics – EnzymixPro (K-99) is a special blend of various enzymes for digestion of sugars, starches, fibers, proteins, and fats.*
ix. *Apex Energetics – GlutenFlam (K-52) is a one-of-a-kind digestive aid that features powerful digestive enzymes to address unintended gluten and casein exposure.*
x. *Standard Process – Dermatrophin PMG is a whole food supplement to support the gut lining.*
xi. *MediHerb – DiGest Forte is a blend herbs for full spectrum digestive support including to help improve HCL production, gastric enzymes, bile, liver metabolism and tone of the GI tract.*

Keep in mind that if you drop a pebble in the water, the greatest impact is the ripple directly next to the surface of the water where the pebble made contact. The same is true with stimulating neural pathways. However, there's always a ripple effect which flows out to benefit more systems in the body that you may be initially trying to help. When you think about stimulating the neural pathways, the more that you can fire at a time, the greater the positive effects that come from that stimulation. The following exercises will help you "fire" the Vagus nerve and keep it active and healthy.

4) At-home Vagus Nerve Stimulation Exercises

Gargling: Gargle for two minutes straight, and I mean gargle like your life depends on it. To accentuate the effect of this stimulation, try fixating on a certain point or part of the wall that's above you. To multiply the positive effects of this even more, do these two things while also doing non-linear complex movements like writing out your name in "air letters" with your free hand or spelling your first and last name.

Ear Lobes: Massaging your outer ear lobes stimulates the Vagus nerve.

The "No No" Exercise: As you focus your attention on a point on the wall, put your feet together and fixate on that point while also rotating your head from right to left *and* humming the "Happy Birthday" song. Then change the exercise by moving your head back and forth as if you're saying "yes yes."

Humming: Humming seems to activate very beneficial parts of the brain that are connected to the Vagus nerve and therefore essential to your gut health.

Gagging: If you're brave enough, try gagging yourself approximately three times until you tear up. Sound intense? It is, but it's one of the best ways to stimulate the Vagus nerve.

If you start to implement these changes, you may begin to notice decreased bloating, gas and diarrhea. You'll notice less brain fog and enjoy improved gut function. We need to see our gut and brain as one because they directly communicate with one another. Now that we've covered your gut, let's move to the next key to solving chronic health problems.

PART THREE

SHARED FOLLOW THROUGH

12

HOW EXAMS HELP YOU HEAL

WHAT IS AN EXAM?

In our clinic, every patient's journey begins with a thorough functional neurological exam. This is a head-to-toe neurological evaluation on you. We do this because we treat every single person as a unique, one-of-a-kind case. Think of the way a detective picks up the trail of a murder case that's gone cold. That's how we approach each person's tangled web of dysfunction. The exam is like cracking open that file and looking at every piece of evidence in a new light.

Many times, exams are used more as a "check off" list for doctors. They're such a rich opportunity for the doctor to gather valuable data about their patient, yet they don't bother to ask enough questions or get the right kind of data needed to really solve the patient's problems. Too often, doctors come in with preconceived notions and they don't put their hands on their patients. Yes, you actually have to touch your patient to do a neurological exam.

In my experience, performing a thorough neurological exam is both an art and a science. The art aspect focuses on how to perform the exam fluidly and in a systematic way that identifies which systems are not functioning properly and are likely damaged. It's also an art form to identify and then assist the most devastated areas of the patient's brain. The science portion comes from all the neurology in classroom learning at the universities as well as textbooks. Most doctors can do the science part. It's the art part that's rare.

I use the same acronym to guide me through every single patient exam, and it's called POPQRST.

> P – Primary complaint. What health issue is having the biggest negative impact on their life? Has anyone else in their family had this issue before?
> O – Onset. When did the symptoms start? And is the primary complaint staying the same or getting worse?
> P – Pain. What provokes the pain and what makes it better?
> Q – Quality of pain. Is there burning, numbness, or tingling?
> R – Radiate. Does the pain radiate out or does it stay local?
> S – Severity. Rank the pain on a scale of 1–10. How bad is it?
> T – Time. What time of day or night is the primary complaint worse?

During this exam, we also test the patient's oxygen levels to determine if they're anemic or not. The body can't heal unless it has the proper supply of oxygen, so this is a crucial first step. We also take their blood pressure (which gives us another hint about their oxygen levels), draw blood and perform intensive blood work, and do glucose testing. All of these tests are getting baseline measurements on the patient's seven keys to health because these keys provide the clues I use to untangle their web of dysfunction and heal their chronic health problems.

During the neurological testing portion of the exam, I use a tuning fork to test the sensitivity of their nervous system. I take the tuning fork, place it on their sternum, and allow them to feel the vibration. That vibration represents a value of 10 and serves as our reference point. Then, I do the same thing but put the tuning fork against their big toe, their thumbs and their shoulders.

Next, I do a two-point discrimination test where I make sure the radial nerve (the nerve which controls sensation in the back of the arm and forearm) is intact and functioning. Then, I test the lower extremities using a two point discrimination test. I check the L-4 saphenous nerve (controls sensation to the inside of the lower leg) and L-5 superficial peroneal nerve (controls the outside of the lower leg). I follow that test with the digit span test where I evaluate the Median nerve which controls the thumb and first and second fingers. I then check Ulnar nerve sensation to part of the ring finger and little finger. Next, I perform the digit span test on the toes via the L-5 superficial peroneal nerve which controls all sensation on the top of the feet as well as all toes (except the small toe which is controlled by the S-1 sural nerve). These tests give me a good indication of how the patient's peripheral nervous system as well as the parietal lobe, located in the back half of the brain, is functioning. Next, I test their reflexes which tells me how well their motor reflexes are responding. Human beings have 10 motor reflexes, and I test all reflexes to see how well their cerebellum, brain and spinal cord are working.

CEREBELLUM TESTS:

After that, I ask them to stand up, if they can, and put their feet together and close their eyes. Next, I'll ask the patient to close their eyes and put their right foot in front of the left foot. Then, I have them switch legs. I follow that exercise up by asking them to alternately lift each leg off the ground and hold it at a 90 degree angle. If your cerebellum is functioning optimally you should be able to maintain each balance/stability test for fifteen seconds. I continue the neurological part of the exam by testing them for smell, fine motor skills, and many more factors that show me the state of their neurological health.

Finger to nose test: I ask the patient to close their eyes and try to place their little finger on the tip of their nose. Fingertip to nose tip.

If they miss, they probably have a decreased functioning cerebellum on the side being tested.

It's important to approach an exam with humility and curiosity because I'm working in the field of probabilities, not absolutes. If you're aspiring to be an accountant or an engineer and seeking absolute answers, this probably is not the field for you. Practically nothing in neurology is absolute. Approaching the patient as if they're a completely new, one-of-a-kind case is the most important mental shift I make every time I prepare to do an exam.

THE FUNDAMENTALS OF AN EFFECTIVE EXAM

When a patient comes into the clinic for an exam, they'll have already filled out their paperwork and we have their blood work results on hand. I start the exam by asking them some questions. Then I move into the primary pillars of executing a great exam.

> Pillar One: Where is the problem? Is it neurological, metabolic or both?
> Pillar Two: How much can we stimulate the system before it fatigues?
> Pillar Three: Do I think I can improve this patient's well being?

Often, the exam reveals new and insightful information that helps us "crack the case." One of my favorite stories is of a young lady who came into the clinic for an exam. She was twenty-one years old and had been a soccer player before her condition forced her to quit sports and drop out of school. She was afflicted with 15–20 seizures per day and had been to all of the major hospitals and experts in the country, yet she was still struggling. Any kind of major stimulation sent her into a seizing fit. If she got out of the car and the sun hit her eyes wrong, she started seizing.

Through neurological testing and the exam, I discovered she had a possible autoimmune disorder, and her oxygen levels were very low.

Her feet and hands were also very cold which meant they weren't getting adequate oxygen. It turned out she had developed autoimmunity against her gut.

I prescribed a treatment plan of Vagal nerve stimulation, the Freedom Metabolic Restore program, brain stimulation therapy, and many other home-based modalities. Once we identified the root cause of her problem, which was the autoimmune condition, we began this treatment protocol that targeted the root cause of her dysfunction. Within four months, she no longer had any seizures. Since then, she re-enrolled in school and wants to become a physical therapist. This is the power of doing the right kind of exam. The clues I found in the neurological exam helped me figure out what part of the body was malfunctioning, and when we addressed the root of the problem, she got her life back.

Another favorite story is of a patient who had been told he needed to move to an assisted living facility because of his poor health and lack of coordination. He initially came in for "frozen" shoulders that wouldn't move his arms above 90 degrees. Through a neurological exam, we discovered the part of the brain that was malfunctioning. We used brain stimulation therapy to activate certain muscle groups to reset the neurological receptors in that part of the body which allowed the brain to recognize and execute the full range of motion. Within four minutes of his first treatment, he went from being able to lift his arms from 90 degrees to lifting them above his head to 180 degrees. From that point, we worked together to heal a whole cascade of chronic health problems that were holding him back and limiting his quality of life. Within nine months of receiving treatment at our clinic, he and his family were back to adventuring. They've since traveled to Yellowstone National Park, Israel, and taken many other big trips.

This is why I treat every single person as a unique, one-of-a-kind case. Every person's tangled web of dysfunction is different and caused by a different combination of dysfunctional processes. The exam is how we open that cold-case file and start to uncover what's going on beneath the surface.

13

OUR PROGRAM

THE PHASES OF DECLINE

The "phases of decline" refer to the stages someone struggling with chronic health problems will experience as their dysfunctional process advances. While this book is ultimately about hope and the encouragement that it is often possible to stop and reverse physical damage and disorders, you also need to take these phases of decline seriously because there is a point of no return. At this point, the body becomes so damaged that it's not possible to regenerate your health to a normal state. Let's take a look at the phases of decline for the three most common maladies I see in my clinic—brain disorders, knee pain, and neuropathy.

PHASES OF DECLINE FOR BRAIN DISORDERS

PHASE ONE: FULL HEALTH

No symptoms expressed at all.

PHASE TWO: EASILY DISMISSIBLE SYMPTOMS

These are things like brain fog that just won't go away, difficulty focusing and concentrating for long periods of time, and a loss of attention to the things you normally enjoy and love. At this point, your brain cells are actually dying, yet most people won't take action, instead choosing to casually dismiss the changes. The patient usually doesn't take responsibility or action, at least not yet.

PHASE THREE/FOUR: RECOGNIZABLE SYMPTOMS

At this stage, things are beginning to progress. You may walk into a room and forget why you walked in there in the first place. Or you may call someone on the phone and forget why you called them. This is an advanced stage of brain degeneration. This is the point where the adult kids may tease their parents about having "old timers" syndrome or say things like "Mom is just losing it…" At this stage, it's very important to filter who you listen to. Your healthcare provider, your kids, your friends, or your spouse may laugh it off, but it's nothing to joke about. At this phase, you must stand up and take responsibility for your health. If you know something isn't right, keep pursuing a solution until you get answers.

PHASE FIVE: THE LIMITATION OF MATTER

At this stage, the brain is degenerated to the point where the person is no longer motivated and simply doesn't have the brain ability to solve their own problems. They no longer see themselves as the problem; instead, everyone else has a problem. When someone reaches this stage, it is very hard and nearly impossible to bring them back. It's a very serious case when someone gets to this stage. It's called "limitation of matter" because at this point, the brain has degenerated so far that it's unable to regenerate and repair to its former state. I don't accept patients for care who are at this stage of degeneration.

COMMON TREATMENTS FOR BRAIN DISORDERS:

These are the common in-clinic treatments that I do for brain-based disorders.

- BrainTap brain fitness – Braintapping is a quick and easy way to optimize your brain's peak potential. Backed by neuroscience, BrainTap is proven to help people with high stress, difficulty sleeping, low energy, and other lifestyle changes.
- Exercise with oxygen therapy – This is simply putting an oxygen mask on the patient and having them ride a stationary bike for twenty minutes while breathing in pure oxygen.
- ReBuilder – This powerful machine helps stimulate proper nerve function.
- Pulse Electro-Magnetic Field (PEMF) machine – This machine is like a battery re-charger for your body. It helps to recharge the cells of the body to the perfect charge to maintain optimal cellular function.
- At-Home Exercises – Vagal stimulation exercises, Freedom Metabolic Restore program, and proper nutritional supplementation.

PHASES OF DECLINE FOR KNEE PAIN

I classify chronic knee pain as anything that has existed for three months or longer. Most of the people who come see me for knee pain have had it for years, if not decades, and can barely walk or get out of a chair. They often have difficulty getting out of bed or off the couch, and their life is severely impacted by their pain. One of the first things I do with every knee pain patient is take x-rays of the knee. We can use regenerative medicine at the clinic, but in order for that treatment to be effective, there has to be a space between the knee joint as seen on the radiograph. The space is important because it means there is still tissue present that can be rehabilitated. If there's no space, they've reached the limitation of matter and have to be referred out for a knee replacement.

I don't accept everyone that comes into the office as a patient. If I do the exam and, based on their results, I don't think I can help them, I refer the patient to a health professional who can better assist them.

However, if the x-ray shows enough spacing in the joint, I may start with a regenerative medicine treatment plan to help them eliminate their chronic pain and regain mobility. Here are some of the solutions that have worked exceptionally well for our knee pain patients.

COMMON TREATMENTS FOR KNEE PAIN:

- The Ergo-Flex Knee-On-Track – This is a machine that decompresses the knee and opens up the joint space, promoting healing and pain relief.
- Oxygen therapy with exercise – I talked about this treatment earlier in the book, but this is simply putting an oxygen mask on the patient and having them ride a stationary bike for twenty minutes while breathing in oxygen.
- ReBuilder – This powerful machine helps stimulate proper nerve function.
- Laser therapy – This treatment decreases inflammation and pain by dilating the capillaries to promote blood flow and encourage the healing properties to access the joint.
- Pulse Electro-Magnetic Field (PEMF) machine – This machine is like a battery re-charger for your body. It helps to recharge the cells of the body to the perfect charge to maintain optimal cellular function.
- NeuroReconnect System – This modality activates the two main receptors of the brain so that they fire into the cerebellum, spinal cord and brain to decrease pain and increase mobility.

PHASES OF DECLINE FOR NEUROPATHY:

Neuropathy patients are usually the most complicated cases because neuropathy can be caused by so many different dysfunctions. These patients often have oxygen problems, glucose problems, and their brain has deteriorated because of a lack of stimulation from their feet. Many people with neuropathy also have erectile or sexual dysfunction.

> Phase One: The feet begin tingling or experiencing a pins and needles sensation.
> Phase Two: Coldness and color changes in the toes and feet.
> Phase Three: The tingling becomes a burning pain.
> Phase Four: Loss of sensation in the legs, feet, toes.

COMMON TREATMENTS FOR NEUROPATHY:

- Blood sugar regulation – I work with the patient to help them balance their blood sugar so their neurological system can stabilize and begin the work of healing.
- Spinal decompression – Many patients with neuropathy have L5 damage so I use decompression therapy to relieve the pressure on that area of the spine.
- Oxygen therapy with exercise – I talked about this treatment earlier in the book, but this is simply putting an oxygen mask on the patient and having them ride a stationary bike for twenty minutes while breathing in oxygen.
- ReBuilder on their feet – This powerful machine helps stimulate proper nerve function.
- Laser therapy – This treatment decreases inflammation and pain by dilating the capillaries to promote blood flow and encourage the healing properties to access the joint.
- Pulse Electro-Magnetic Field (PEMF) machine – This machine is like a battery re-charger for your body. It helps to recharge the cells of the body to the perfect charge to maintain optimal cellular function.
- NeuroReconnect System – This modality activates the two main receptors of the brain so that they fire into the cerebellum, spinal cord and brain to decrease pain and increase mobility.

- BrainTap brain fitness – Braintapping is a quick and easy way to optimize your brain's peak potential. Backed by neuroscience, BrainTap is proven to help people with high stress, difficulty sleeping, low energy, and other lifestyle changes.
- Metabolic Care – Freedom Metabolic Restore program and proper nutritional supplementation.

CUSTOM MADE

A truly custom, one-of-a-kind healthcare program will impact your health in a way you've never experienced before because it is created uniquely for you. I don't accept everyone for care. If someone isn't fully committed, they're too neurologically damaged, or they're too far degenerated, I'm not going to take them for care and waste their time or money. When I accept someone for care, I make them a promise that I'm on this journey with them, and we're in it to win it. I will exhaust every option I know in order to optimize their recovery. However, we both need to have realistic expectations. If their expectations are beyond what I can give them, we need to realign. I'm always going to under promise and over-deliver, and sometimes tough love requires telling people the truth that they don't want to hear.

A custom healthcare program to heal your chronic disease always comes as a result of a thorough and effective neurological examination process, and it always addresses all aspects of your metabolic and neurological health. However, the truth is that if they don't follow the program I prescribe them, they're probably not going to get the results they want. No one is going to care more about your health than you. If you don't want to be well, live vibrantly, and leave a legacy, no one is going to do it for you. I'm totally committed to the patient, but they need to be "all in" too.

14

A POSITIVE OUTCOME IS OUR GOAL

In the first interaction I have with any patient, I want to confirm first and foremost that they are in the right place. Not every person that walks into our practice is meant to be a patient. Some need surgery, some want a "quick fix," some aren't ready to take control of their health and their life, and some won't invest financially in themselves. Those that are ready to change their life and willing to invest their time and resources into getting results are in the right place. Our team will make their positive outcome our goal.

When seeing a new doctor, most patients are nervous and unsure if they have made the right choice. We provide an environment that helps patients feel welcome, reassures them, and begins to restore hope. We are a family practice with Christian values and our clinic is set up to feel inviting, warm, and encouraging. Even the music we play throughout the office is uplifting and prompts healthy choices. For instance, we play satellite radio without commercials because we don't want our patients to be bombarded with ads that encourage them to eat and drink things that aren't part of their care plan. We even refer to the patient's paperwork as "paper *fun*."

The environment and care we provide is only made possible because of the team, the family of providers we have cultivated. The benefits of our integrated clinic enable us to keep treatment plans shorter and speed up recovery time because we are all working together under one roof. The tools and support are already there for the patient so they can work through a plan faster. With multiple disciplines under the same roof, there are a lot of options available, and we are able to fit the care according to the patient's specific needs. We are also able to automatically provide a patient with a second opinion.

All of this leads to a successful doctor-patient relationship. It requires teamwork, communication, and a willingness to set realistic goals. But none of that works unless we first care about each person that walks through our doors. That care creates mutual trust and ensures that both parties engage in the process that leads to the life-changing effects of our care.

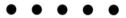

Beginning the journey back to optimized health can be hard, but we want our clinic to be a respite. It's still a process, but there's no reason that the journey can't be fun and hope-filled along the way. That's the ultimate goal, a positive outcome that helps a patient feel better, improves their health, and changes their life. Reaching this goal takes time and requires the patient and doctors to commit to the process. I know the process has worked when the patient gets their positive outcome. In turn, when a patient trusts us with their family members or friends (which happens often), I am affirmed that it is about more than just a single positive outcome—it's about life-changing results.

I've seen many life-changing outcomes over the years.

For example, I remember a father bringing his daughter in to see us. She was a cheerleader and had fallen from the top of the pyramid. When she came in, her arm was trembling like a Parkinson's patient. We did a thorough exam, and as I began to adjust her, I simply bent her head over my hand in a certain direction and her tremor stopped.

It took several treatments before we were able to get the tremor to go away completely. But in that single moment, she knew, her dad knew, and I knew this would change her life. There's no telling how long she would have dealt with that tremor, how much it would have affected her life in school and her involvement in cheerleading, but because her dad trusted us, I was able to give her a positive outcome.

• • • • •

When I reflect on the growth of the Freedom Health Centers family, I see the lessons my parents taught me growing up: integrity, hard work, and a constant desire to keep learning. It was that ability and desire to keep learning that ultimately led me to recognize the importance of Dr. Andy Barlow's work. With his guidance, we have helped those with advanced neurological issues, auto-immunity, and brain-based disorders. Health is a journey, and unfortunately, there will always be new chronic issues waiting on the horizon. But I know that we will be ready for whatever comes next because we are always ready to learn more. Growing up, I always knew I wanted to help as many people as I could, and with each new implementation of testing and care we achieve that goal.

TAKE ACTION

I encourage you to ask yourself these questions:

- How long have you lived with your pain/issue?
- How long have you tried to lose weight?
- How long have you thought there was no hope for you?
- How long are you going to wait before you seek a better outcome?

If your answers can be summed up with the words, "I've been living with this issue for too long, and I'm not going to wait another minute to do something about it," then I would love to hear from you!

All the best to you!

Dr. Todd A. Molski, D.C.
Freedom Health Centers
972-542-3300
www.freedomhealthcenters.com